MW00411795

CINDY CROSBY *and* THOMAS DEAN

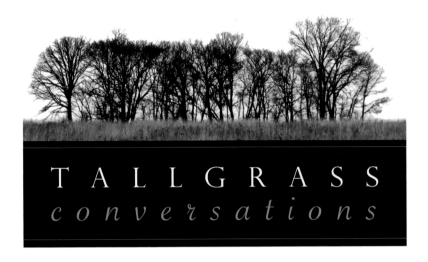

# TALLGRASS
## *conversations*

IN SEARCH OF
THE PRAIRIE SPIRIT

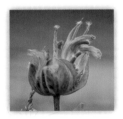

Tom:

*for Susan, Nathaniel, and Sylvia*

Cindy:

*for Jeff*

First Edition

ISBN 9781948509060
Library of Congress Control Number: Available upon request

Ice Cube Press, LLC (Established 1991)
205 N Front Street
North Liberty, Johnson County, Iowa, 52317, USA
www.icecubepress.com steve@icecubepress.com

The paper used in this publication meets the minimum requirements of the American National Standard for Information Sciences—Permanence of Paper for Printed Library Materials, ANSI Z39.48-1992.

Design by Cindy Kiple
cindykiple@gmail.com

# CONTENTS

# INTRODUCTION

*Thomas Dean*

We are always embedded in the land we dwell upon. In practical terms, our physical bodies are dependent on a functioning ecosystem, so our inescapable obligation of environmental care is to our own benefit as well as that of the health, well-being, and integrity of the living earth. But when we are truly home in the world, the other aspects of our beings—spiritual, aesthetic, emotional—are also inextricably entwined with nature. For those of us in much of the continent's middle land, our natural home is the tallgrass prairie.

As I mention in one essay in this collection, despite a life lived entirely in the Midwest, my awareness of—and love for—the prairie came only in adulthood. I don't recall one mention of bluestem or spiderwort in all of my schooling. As an Iowan transplanted from Illinois, I live and have lived in arguably the most altered land in the world. As a child, my understanding of prairie, if the word was invoked at all, meant something more abstract, such as "flat Midwest that you plant corn on."

Obviously, "prairie" doesn't mean that at all. And while I have learned much as an adult about the native grasses, forbs, animals, waters, and soil of the land I live on, I have also come to understand how much prairie is part of who I am—my identity, my spirit, my aesthetic sense, my emotions, and much more. Cultivating a land ethic, as Aldo Leopold would call it, to care for that land clearly involves communicating with others. Drawing out our under-standings of self and culture does as well. The arts of conversation, then, are essential to building a vibrant relationship not only with other people but the place that is our home. To be in search of the prairie spirit here in this place on earth means to engage in tallgrass conversations.

When I asked Cindy Crosby if she would like to collaborate on a book about the prairie, we were in the midst of a conversation, appropriately enough (an exchange about her previous prairie book). Conversation has always been at the heart of this book's concept and origin, even before we settled on *Tallgrass Conversations* as a title. If we think of it broadly as an exchange that brings two or more entities together and dynamically creates something new, conversation is perhaps our greatest hope not only for healing the rifts in human understanding but also for restoring and reinspiring our relationship with the natural world that is our home.

In this book, conversation works on multiple levels. I have admired Cindy's words and photos in her *Tuesdays in the Tallgrass* blog, and I have had a burgeoning interest in photography in addition to my work as a writer, so I suggested we publish a book that brings our individual prairie voices and prairie eyes together. Cindy and I have different backgrounds, different writing voices, and different photographic perspectives, yet we both bring them to bear on our love and advocacy for the tallgrass prairie. We thought bringing together these differences, rooted in common ground, could yield yet more new understandings of the prairie and inspire others to enter tallgrass conversations of their own.

On individual levels, our own writings and photographs converse symbiotically in this book, with the hope that bringing two expressive forms together will create an artistic whole greater than the sum of their parts. But more importantly, Cindy and I intended to converse with each other, to have our words and images play off of one another. Our ultimate aspiration is that we inspire you, our readers, to understand and enrich your experience of the prairie in ways you haven't before, whether you are a naturalist, conservationist, writer, artist, activist, environmentalist, outdoor enthusiast . . . however you define yourself in relation to the prairie. We also hope that you will be inspired to engage in your own tallgrass conversations, bringing your personal multiple expressive forms together and then maybe exchanging them with others. In so doing, we hope you will not only see the prairie anew but also stretch your artistic talents, which need not require years and years of training or a fortune in equipment (both my and Cindy's cameras are relatively simple).

Prairie is among the most altered and threatened ecosystems in the world. At the same time, our natural world is our first and most profound home. Care of the world is always essential, and care arises from conversation. We invite you to join us on this journey of care and inspiration through your own tallgrass conversations.

January 2019
Iowa City, Iowa

# INTRODUCTION

*Cindy Crosby*

*I*'m a big fan of stories. So, when I moved to the Chicago suburbs more than twenty years ago and saw my first tallgrass prairie (or at least, the first prairie I recognized as such), I wanted to know its history. Its flora. Its community of insects, birds, and mammals. I wanted to hear the story the prairie has to tell.

Slowly, over time—evenings spent sitting in the grasses, mornings spent hiking the trails, volunteer workdays—I came into conversation with the prairie. I took prairie classes and became a steward. Pulled weeds, collected seeds. Planted a prairie patch in my suburban backyard. Began teaching prairie classes. Talked nonstop about prairie to patient friends and family members. I went back to school to get my master's degree in natural resources so I would understand more about the beautiful landscape called home in the Midwest. Began writing a blog about prairie, *Tuesdays in the Tallgrass*; penning books about my journeys with prairie. Each season, as I learned about, walked, and listened to the prairie, it told me a little more of its story.

It's a story of love and loss. Hard work and sweat. Disappointment and triumph. Diversity. A struggle against brush and trees. A triumph of a few small parcels of original prairie hanging on in the middle of golf courses, farm fields, and subdivisions. It's a tale of how the land was once viewed by people. A place to be conquered. Grocery store. A place for development and agriculture. Apothecary. A barren wasteland. A place for research. A place to meditate. The landscape of home.

The Nature Conservancy calls the North American tallgrass prairie a more threatened ecosystem than the Amazon rainforest. The prairie is irreplaceable. Who knows what keys the remaining prairie may hold for our future? So many mysteries are still in these plants, the soil, the grassland community! To unlock some of the prairie's secrets requires that we have an actual prairie to learn from. And this is where this book comes in.

John T. Price says in the introduction to his edited collection of essays, *The Tallgrass Prairie Reader*, that a lack of writing about grasslands has given us "another kind of extinction." Price believes that the effort to understand and combat the destruction of tallgrass prairie "must also take place in the hearts and minds of our citizens, the realm under the purview of literature and art."

As coauthors of this book on tallgrass prairie, Tom and I want to see this change. We need more writers and artists; poets and photographers, documenting what's left of this amazing landscape. We need to raise awareness of what was lost—not to mourn, although that is a part of it—but to connect people's hearts and minds with our prairie restorations and remnants and to prevent further loss. We need you to partner with us in sharing the prairie through words, images, and experiences.

Writes Gerould Wilhelm in his book (with coauthor Laura Rericha), "Given the fragile nature of landscapes with high natural quality, there is no substitute for their preservation and proper management. No amount of *de novo* restoration can obviate concern over their passing." We can't replace what is lost. Not completely. Remnant prairie functions in a way we can't replicate through planting prairie.

But we can educate ourselves about what we are losing. We can care for what remains. We can continue to plant prairie, then research, paint, write about, and ensure tallgrass prairie is a part of future conversations about development, agriculture, and conservation.

In this book, Tom and I both have a passion for prairie in our respective parts of the region; Tom in Iowa, me in Illinois. We also appreciate savanna—open oak woodland systems with their own associated plants—another ecosystem different from but often associated with a prairie. We include some essays, photos, and references to savanna as well as prairie throughout the book. But the way we see tallgrass prairie and savanna is as varied as our photos and our essays. Each of us responded to words in the prairie conversation differently, just as a conversation between two people about the same idea can hold various perspectives. We hope you'll enjoy seeing the various ways we invite you to think about some of these words and images that showcase the prairie spirit.

You, too, will see these prairie images through your own lens of knowledge, relationship, and experiences in new and different ways than we do. The more facets of prairie we can understand through these different lenses, the greater chance there is for preservation in the future.

Consider this book your invitation to the conversation. As you get to know prairie, or deepen your relationship with an already familiar landscape, we want to offer you a chance to add your voice to the conversation. When you are done reading and sharing this book with your friends and family, we hope you'll find you've made a connection of the heart with the tallgrass prairie. It has a lot to say to you.

Don't let reading about prairie be enough. Find tallgrass prairies wherever you live or visit—in your community, your region, your state. Then go and see them for yourselves. Prairies survive—from those small one-acre plots tucked into old cemeteries to the large twenty-thousand-plus-acre Midewin National Tallgrass Prairie. They are waiting for you. Go see them. Listen to their stories. And then, tell everyone you know about them in whatever way you can. Through words. Through experiences. Through photographs and paintings and textile work and poetry and articles and literature.

The prairie has much to say to you. Come to the prairie with an open mind and an open heart. It's up to you to keep the tallgrass prairie dialogue going for future generations. Welcome to the conversation.

January 2019
Glen Ellyn, Illinois

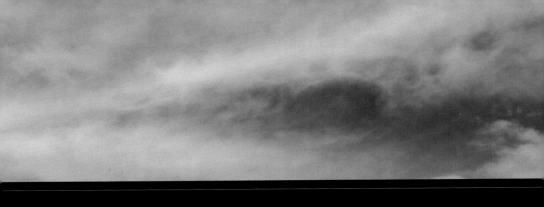

*the spirit of*

# OPENING

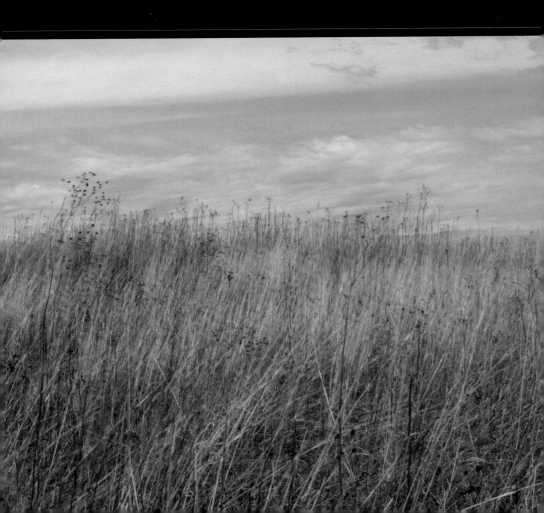

# PATH

*Thomas Dean*

The path to prairie is patience. It cannot be apprehended in a panoramic view, in close study of each plant or animal, or in a single encounter. The path to prairie takes a lifetime to traverse. To enter prairie is a lifelong commitment.

The path to prairie is awe. Without accepting awe, madness may ensue. Legend has it that some European pioneers went insane in the vastness of the sea of grass. Did they fail to revere a horizontal immensity?

The path to prairie is humility, sibling to awe. Within the prairie's vast beauty and mystery, we must accept our smallness, set aside our arrogant dominion, know that even in the presence of the least petal and the slimmest grass blade, we are but humble guests of the grassland.

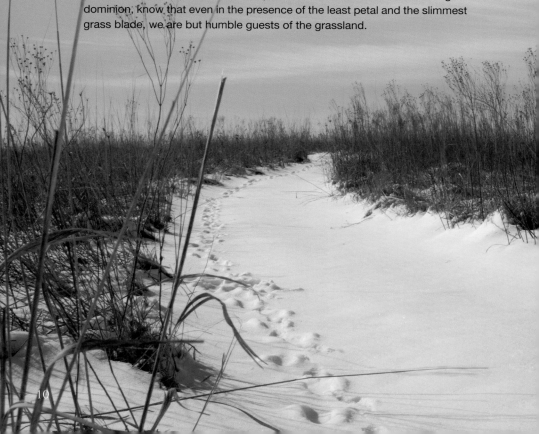

The path to prairie is understanding the unseen. We celebrate the beauty of wildflowers, the majesty of grasses, the fleeting beauty of birds and insects, the stateliness of bison and elk. But we must know most prairie is concealed, underground. The essence of prairie, the life-giving force, is the deep roots that hold soil, deliver water, and feed the subterranean biome. We cannot view prairie's dark beauty and animating energy. If we dig to do so, we destroy them.

The path to prairie is centeredness. We must fix our minds and bodies within our selves, cast off distractions and artifice, or we will fail to perceive, sense, and comprehend the minuteness and the totality of prairie. Missing that, we miss the spirit, the *genius loci*, perhaps the soul of the tallgrass.

The path to prairie is openness. In centering ourselves, we activate the full spectrum of perception, opening our sight, hearing, smell, and touch to the vast variety of life abounding about us. When we are open, we can shift our discernment gracefully from the delicate windflower to the broad expanse of bluestem. When our senses are fully open, we are prepared to receive the earth story the prairie can share with us, a story that leads us to ever-greater gifts.

The earth story is a path we can never complete. The path to prairie is endless. The path to prairie is timeless.

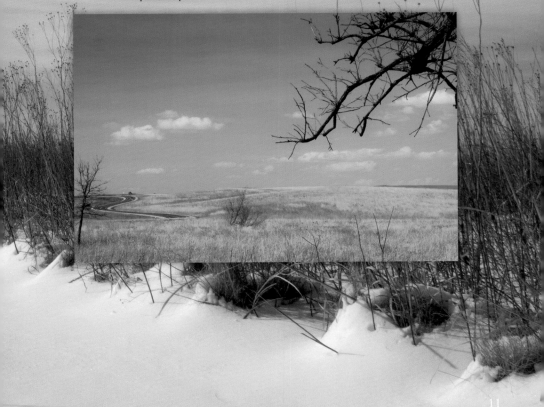

*Cindy Crosby*

*I*'ve been a rule-follower much of my life. If there was a path you were expected to stay on, I was quick to do so.

Here's what the prairie taught me when I first encountered it in my late thirties: leave the path.

I've found following a well-worn path is easy. Doing what you are supposed to. Not upsetting the status quo. Often, there are signs telling you what you are seeing. How to understand what you see. What to do about it.

Sure, the path can be pretty narrow in places, but there's comfort in treading the same well-worn grooves that others have left for you to follow. Look straight ahead. No deviations.

Leaving the path is a bit frightening. Rather than following the same journey made by others, you are creating your own trajectory. Thinking your own thoughts. Going into the unknown. Coming to your own conclusions.

It's easy to doubt yourself. There is that little voice that tells you that you don't know enough. The shaming voice—"What are you doing over there? Get back on that path!" After all, isn't what has worked for so many people good enough for you?

Yes, I like the interpretive panels—those signs along the path with information about a prairie—one of my many jobs in life has been to create them. I also love field guides. They help me orient myself and learn from others. There is collective wisdom in the past, good information for the journey.

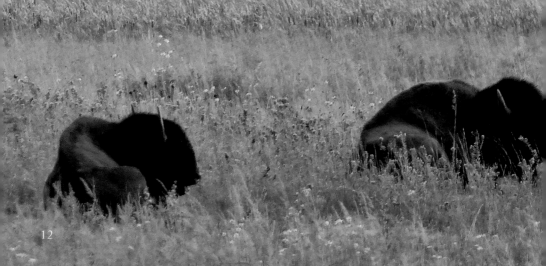

There is only so much, however, you can learn from books and signs and other people. At some point you have to internalize it. Learn with your heart. Walk into something new.

So one day, you go. Step into the unknown. And find yourself drawn in.

Chasing dragonflies required me to move me off the prairie paths. And as I did, I found more than dragonflies. So many delights! Over here, the violet sorrel. Look at this! American burnet, *Sanguisorba canadensis*! One time, I discovered an eastern prairie fringed orchid. On another hike, I found myself in a virtual constellation of shooting star.

There is a sense of openness when you go off-trail. No signs to interpret what you are seeing. Your sense of wonder is on high alert. What discovery will you make next?

By stepping off the path that others chose for me, I found a new perspective on places I loved. And in doing so, I learned more about myself.

And yes. There are places I visited that asked me to stay on the path. I did what I was asked, out of care for the prairie there. Some areas are so fragile, so delicate, that we respect them by watching where we put our hiking boots. We put the greater good ahead of our own desires.

But in other, wilder places, where the paths are optional, I venture out. I've turned my ankle a few times. Fallen down. Gotten bit by mosquitoes, brushed off ticks. One time I came to what I thought was an uncrossable chasm. It took me a long time to make my way across it, and when I did, I was scratched, bruised, and exhausted. But I eventually found my way to the other side.

And isn't that worth the risk?

In "The Journey," poet Mary Oliver wrote "One day, you finally knew what you had to do, and began. . . ."

Go ahead. Step off the path.

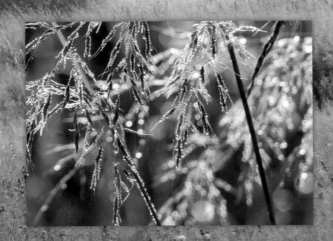

# POSSIBILITIES

*Cindy Crosby*

*W*hen the sandhill cranes pass through Illinois I know it's time to burn. The prescribed fires we set mimic the natural cycle of lightning fires that once torched the tallgrass prairies and kept encroaching trees and brush at bay. Native Americans, who also fired the prairies to drive wild game and entice it to feed upon the new growth, no longer spark the tallgrass. So instead, I and about twenty-five others suit up in yellow slickers, pull on leather gloves and safety glasses, then with our team of prescribed burn members, go out to lay siege to the prairie.

The fire moves fast. Flames roar, consuming dried grasses, wildflower husks, and everything in their path. The flashes of light, the sound of the flames are intense. Dramatic. Then—it's suddenly over. How quickly what has taken months to grow is destroyed! Erased. Seemingly lost.

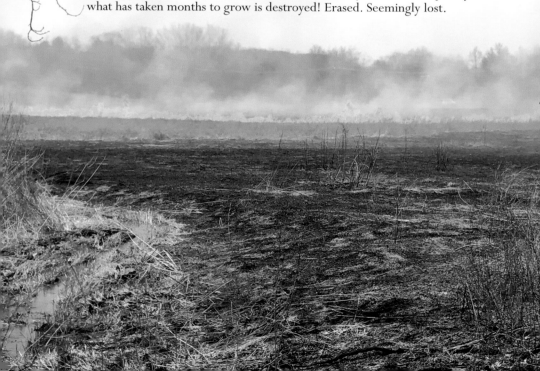

To the uninitiated, this is devastation of the worst sort. But those of us who help manage restoration know that the fires are necessary. Without them, the prairies would eventually vanish in Illinois.

Ashes to ashes, dust to dust. What can a "ground zero" promise us about tomorrow?

Hiking the smoking landscape of the Schulenberg Prairie after the burn, I feel the crunch of tiny mammal bones under my boots. I see the detritus of items lost the previous year: a charred cell phone, a weeding tool left by a prairie volunteer, a bottle tossed out from a car on the road running adjacent.

The landscape is reduced to nothing but ashes, skeletons, and litter.

And yet.

A warm front moves through. Rain drenches the prairie. A sleight of hand occurs. More sunshine. A few weeks go by. What was recently dry, charred, and ashen is a fuzz of emerald. Ponds of rainwater reflect the now-blue sky. The black ash left by the prescribed fire warms the ground, and now hundreds of thousands of grass blades needle their way up from

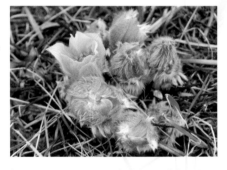

the ruins. Prairie dropseed hummocks, round bumps on the surface of the prairie, are furred with green. The tiny lime yucca-like leaves of rattlesnake master push up in tiny patches along the trails.

I walk, and I look, and I wonder. I gently touch the new leaves in their kaleidoscope of shapes, sizes, and colors. *Welcome back. Welcome back. Welcome back.*

During the fire, the growing points of the prairie perennials were safely tucked underground. The fires nipped a few emergents. But as the sun heats the charred ground, the warmth coaxes the prairie plants to grow again.

Each season in the tallgrass brings repetition, building on what was there the season before. Each season is a new beginning.

Along a craggy outcrop, I carefully hunt for what I know I have seen before. There! Tucked into the scorched rocks I find them: one, two, three early-blooming pasque flowers blossoming in one clump. Their pale, pale lavender petal-like sepals are almost invisible against the stones.

I fall to my knees in the mud. Somehow this trio of blooms has escaped the flames of a late spring burn. The pasque flower's scientific name, *Pulsatilla patens*, refers to the way the open blooms pulsate in the wind.

Its common name, from Latin, means "Easter."

*Thomas Dean*

*S*pring was much delayed, with several snowstorms and weeks of below-average temperatures plaguing Iowa in April. But finally the pattern broke, and the jet stream allowed more persistent southern breezes into the state. On the first warm Saturday, my wife, Susan, and I just had to take the dogs out for a prairie walk.

The winter prairie is dormant, but it has its own character, a presence that to me is more about itself in the moment than about the new growth to come weeks and months later. The silence, the wind, even the previous year's death, still present in the brittle stalks and stems, are of a unique kind, the end of the life cycle. Yet shifts and changes continue subtly throughout the cold time. When I walk the winter prairie, I am in its present time, not its future.

As a living ecosystem, the prairie grows, dies, and metamorphoses every moment of every day. But as we walk our dogs through the grass trails of the Hoover Prairie and welcome the fresh breezes of this first warm April day, we pass the dry remnants of what now seems like a prairie past, *last* year's prairie. We see a few tiny shoots of green emerging from the ground, but I don't yet fully sense them as the new prairie coming alive. This prairie at this moment — this one brief, singular moment in time — is the prairie of possibilities.

Will the spiderwort spread? Will the milkweed be more abundant and attract more monarchs this year? Will the meadowlarks decline further as predicted? Not even the hint of an answer has emerged today — today it is all and only possibility.

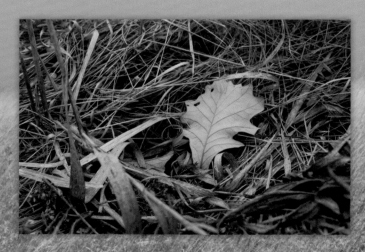

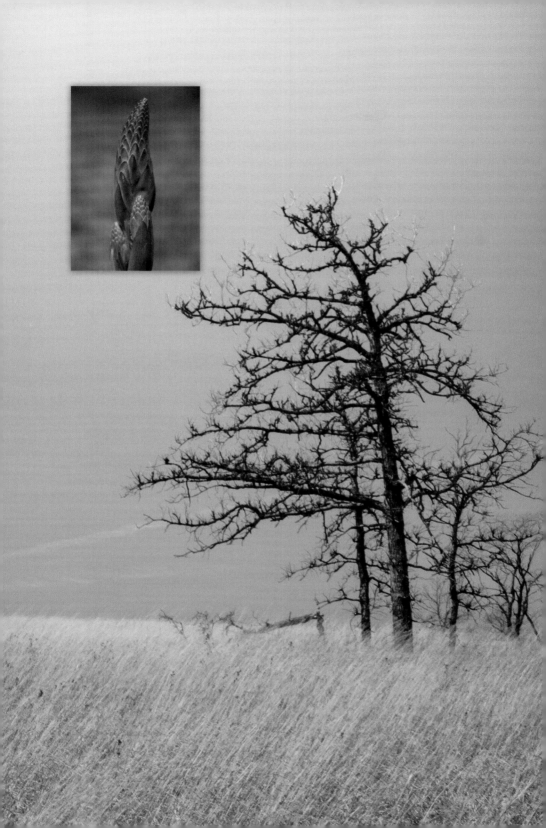

# WORDS

*Cindy Crosby*

While hiking an unfamiliar prairie, I come to a stream limned with ice. The bridge spanning the waterway is gone. *Hmmm.* My choices are simple. I can turn back. Hop from slick rock to slick rock. Or wade the shallows to the other side and get my feet wet.

Reluctantly, I choose the path of least resistance and retrace my path. The rest of the prairie will have to wait for another day's exploration, better footwear, or the bridge repair.

As one who seeks to know new places more intimately, I'm reminded that the loss of bridges—connecting points—matters. As a writer, I get that as well. Words are bridges. They have the capability to connect us to places—and to dynamic ideas. They elicit memory. They provoke action. They stimulate emotion. They are a springboard for the imagination.

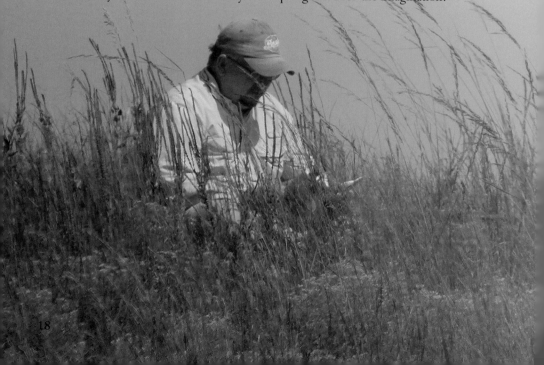

How many times has a parent told you, "Her first word was —"? Or a grieving person, "His last words were —"? Words are significant! Our ancestors also knew the importance of words. The First Amendment notes, "Congress shall make no law respecting an establishment of religion, or prohibiting the free exercise thereof; or abridging the freedom of speech, or of the press." Words matter. Losing words matters.

When we lose particular words about place, we lose part of our collective memory. These words comprise a slice of our identity. They are the language of the place in which we live. More specifically, when we lose prairie-related vocabulary, we break links that join us to the tallgrass, specific identifiers that bind us to a place.

Words are one way we give human voice to a land that speaks in prairie dropseed, bobolinks, and dung beetles. Naming things brings them to our attention, just as learning the name of someone we meet makes them more memorable, more "real" to us.

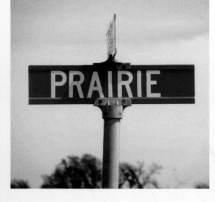

When we learn the name for a particular sedge or a specific bee, we can visualize it, even when it isn't in front of us. In a time when tallgrass prairie and grasslands are dubbed "the world's most imperiled ecosystem" by the Nature Conservancy, to lose any of the names that belong to prairie is to lose some of our momentum in cherishing and caring for grasslands.

We're lazy. We don't have enough time, do we? It's easier to use nondescriptive, bland words that trip easily off the tongue. *Ecosystem. Landscape. Grasses. Plants. Bugs.* I use many of them myself! But too many generalities and the prairie becomes a blur, a nonentity.

There is rhythm and motion in the prairie vocabulary, joy in the particulars. Delight in the common names: Canada wild rye. Regal fritillary. Hoary puccoon. Cream wild indigo. Try saying some of the scientific names out loud: *Bison bison.* (That double whammy! Like a drumbeat.) Or *Monarda fistulosa. Spiza americana*, the dicksissel, a bird whose song has provided the soundtrack for many a prairie hike. Let these descriptive words roll off your tongue: *Mesic. Mollisols. Loess.*

Speak the words. Keep them in front of people. It's a fragile hold we have on these words. Don't let anyone tell you otherwise.

Words bring light into the world; help shine understanding into dark corners. Words of color and sound. Words of hope. Words of restoration. Words of promise.

Specific words matter. Let's use them.

*Thomas Dean*

One of the most important portrayals of the preagricultural tallgrass is Hamlin Garland's *Boy Life on the Prairie*, an 1899 fictionalized autobiography of growing up on an Iowa farm from 1869 to 1881. The story of young "Lincoln Stewart" on the Iowa frontier includes eyewitness scenes of the uncultivated prairie. Euro-American writers often struggled to find words to describe the previously unseen vast grassland, and Garland's language often did not stray far from typical nineteenth-century notions.

The prairie spectacle was so overwhelming that Lincoln's first encounter is cast in otherworldly terms: "It was as though he had suddenly been transported into another world, a world where time did not exist; where snow never fell, and the grass waved forever under a cloudless sky. A great awe fell upon him as he looked, and he could not utter a word." Even though young Lincoln strains to find earthly language to describe his new grassland home, his words also reflect the historical loss of the prairie before he can barely apprehend it.

The young boy's eyes gaze away from town toward where "the unclaimed prairie rolled," implying the land is there for humans to wrest for their own purposes.

Further, Garland's words tie Lincoln's adventures with friends on the "unclaimed" prairie to the era's disturbing attitudes toward Native peoples, referring to the boys' exploits as "return[ing] to the primitive" and "the freedom of the savage." When returning home "to the warmly lighted kitchen and to mother," the day has "united . . . the pleasures of both civilization and barbarism." As the book progresses, the phrase, typical of its time, "the vanishing prairie" is invoked, echoing the simultaneously romanticized and deliberately exterminated "noble savage" or "vanishing Indian" of the late nineteenth century.

Garland's story seems to view the "vanishing" grassland as regrettable but inevitable. At the end of the book, Lincoln returns to his frontier home at age twenty-four to find "every acre . . . cultivated" and "no sign of the prairie grass." He and his friend Rance ride their horses many miles to find any "vacant land." When they stumble upon a vestigial "slip of prairie sod" along a railway track, Lincoln throws himself into the tiny remnant, yet resigned to the "inexorable march of civilization" that has left virtually no prairie unplowed.

Fortunately, most no longer see the prairie as an otherworldly landscape, and we've put words such as "unclaimed"—let alone "primitive," "savage," and "barbaric"—behind us. Many—hopefully most—who appreciate the prairie realize that the "march of civilization" was a choice and not "inexorable," and that we must not be fatalistic about an inevitably "vanishing" prairie. These days when we talk about prairie, we're instead apt to use words such as "sustainability," "ecosystem," and "restoration."

Even so, such terminology has a rather clinical ring to it. In a world of climate destabilization and accelerating ecological loss, such concepts are vital. But to me, prairie is more than a system, and my motivation to care for and experience it goes beyond just sustaining it. I think other words are important to invoke and explore, too, as we make prairie part of our lives—words such as "joy," "majesty," "mystery," "wonder," and "home." Those are the words I wish to embrace in my tallgrass conversations.

# HOME

*Thomas Dean*

The savanna called me home. In a retreat called "The Great Conversation: Nature and the Care of the Soul" with Belden Lane at Prairiewoods Franciscan Spirituality Center, we were asked to seek out a teacher among nature's beings on the ecospirituality center's land. As happens every time I visit Prairiewoods, the small savanna of six swamp white oaks drew me to enter into council with them.

The savanna is humanity's home. The grassland dotted with scattered groups of trees is the original African terrain where our ancestors roamed, ran, and dwelled with the creatures of the earth. When shown pictures of various landscapes and ecosystems, people still tend to choose savanna as the most attractive, the one they identify with most. As a species, we are inexorably drawn to savanna, as I was once again at Prairiewoods on a cold March day. The savanna grounds us in fields of grasses that spread below, around, and beyond us. Most definitions of home speak of a sense of familiarity, safety, security, identity. No other landscape speaks of home to us more than savanna.

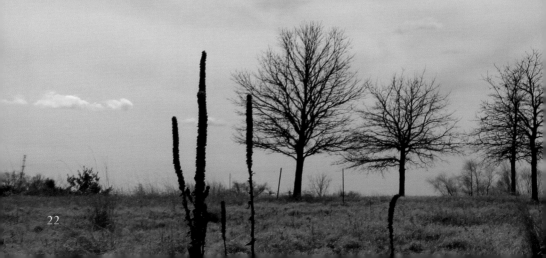

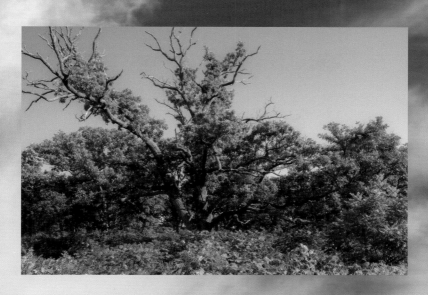

We are also drawn to savanna's enigma. It is an edge landscape, a transition between horizon of grasses and vertex of canopy. It is shadow and light playing invitations across a threshold to mystery, drawing us into both the boundless unknown and the center of wholeness, just as home does.

The prairie had been burned that spring at Prairiewoods, so entering the circle of trees was easy. I was able to approach, honor, and converse with the six oaks in ways I had not been able before. I heard gratitude for the life-giving fire Prairiewoods' staff had given to the oaks' companions — soil and plants beneath and beyond its canopy of branches. I heard an invitation to touch one of the tree's rough, hard trunks, to close my eyes and to feel the turning of the earth. I heard their plea to stop cutting and poisoning,

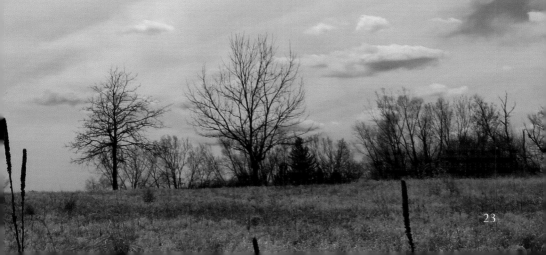

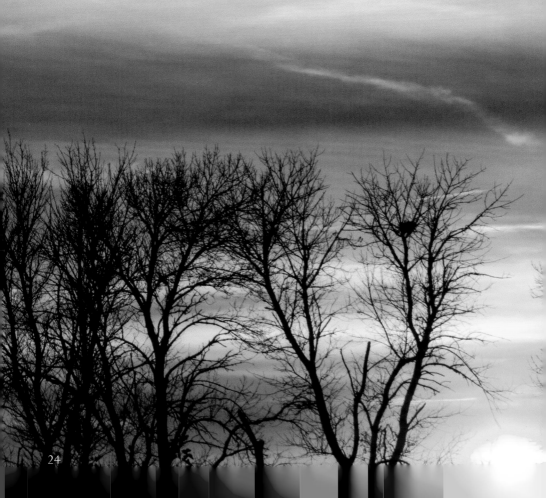

which has made the oak savanna an even more endangered landscape in our state than the prairie itself. Perhaps most importantly, the sturdy sentinels, spreading their broad branches wide above me, told me they were a bound family rooted in ground and held together in this place. And they were also holding me here, ever present for me as I venture out into the open spaces and possibilities of prairie. They are nature's family, always there for me to return home.

Here in the middle lands of Iowa, prairie and savanna once rolled before us for hundreds of miles and millions of acres. Yet we have laid waste to them. We have laid waste to home. Why humanity destroys its own home is perhaps the greatest bewilderment of our modern existence.

Savanna and prairie root us in place, challenge us to cross their mysterious edges, and invite us to return always—but also to be more mindful of the care and honor we are obliged to provide. Savanna and prairie are where I—where we—always return. Savanna and prairie are home.

## Cindy Crosby

The real estate market on the May prairie is booming. Everywhere I look, critters pair up, make homes, and settle down to raise their families.

The spiders find wood betony blooms the perfect structures to sling their webs of tensile strength silks. Burly bison, weighing a thousand pounds or more, throw their first calves. Rough-haired and knock-kneed. Close by, diminutive thirteen-lined ground squirrels look for love. They nestle in the tallgrass together, then, alarmed at any sudden sound, pop down a tunnel. Newborns will arrive in less than a month.

In wetland lodges, beavers welcome their newborn kits. Their waterfront property is the perfect launching pad for the summer's adventures. The first dragonflies and damselflies emerge from their underwater nurseries. Green darners (*Anax junius*) lead the way. If you are patient—and lucky enough—you will see the dragonflies emerge in their teneral stage, clinging to grass blades over the water. Not quite nymph. Not quite adult. Slowly, their fragile wings fill and pump open. Colors and patterns sharpen into focus. The newly minted flyers warm to their new lives. Disappear into the sunshine.

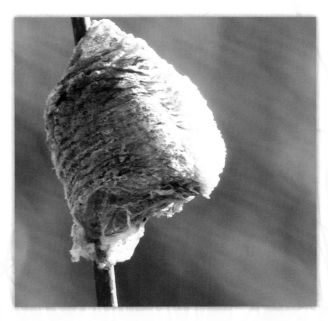

The prairie is suddenly full of sound. Spring peepers, chorus frogs, and an American toad or two call from the ephemeral ponds. Warblers sing from the prairie's edges, happy to be home after their long migrations from the south. Grassland birds craft nests, full of potential birdsong.

A warm breeze stirs. The young grasses, less than knee high, wave in the wind. Native bees and pollinators hum enthusiastically from flower to flower on high alert. *Does this bloom have nectar? Or this one?* They pack pollen on each side like tourists hoisting orange suitcases and move their "bags" from flower to flower. Queen bumblebees search out likely spots for ground nests, ready to set up housekeeping when the right location is found.

It's spring on the prairie. The season of making a home. The season of *coming* home.

To our landscape of home.

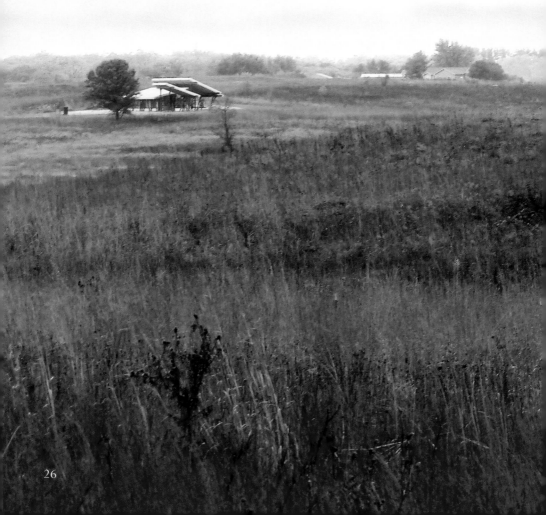

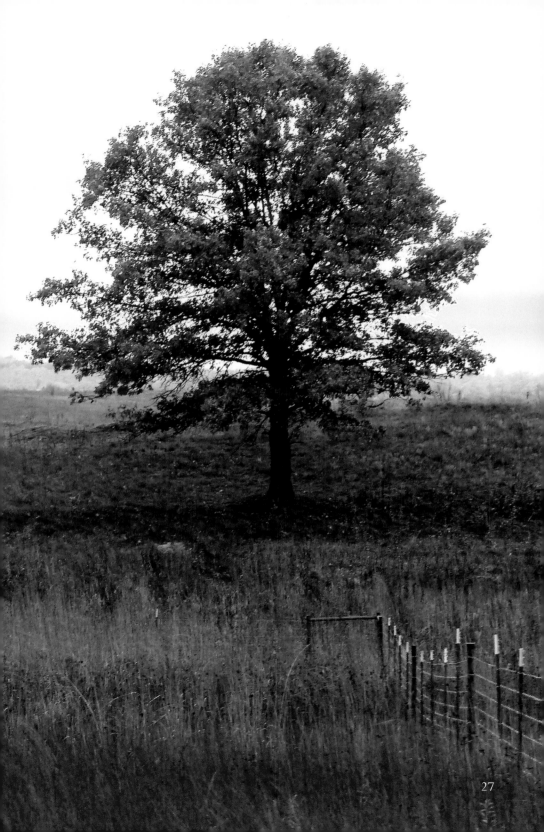

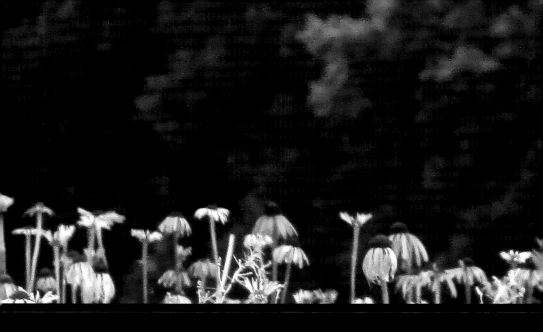

# the spirit of
# AWARENESS

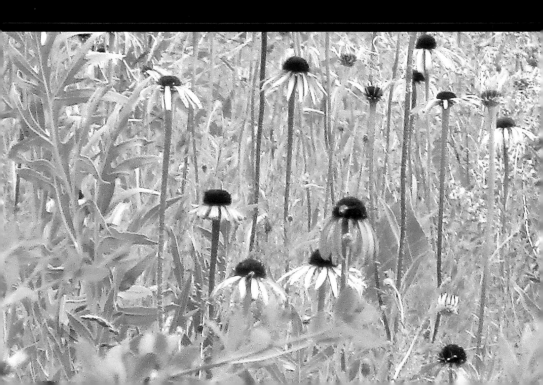

*conversation five*

# LOSS

*Cindy Crosby*

It's sunset. The small patch of prairie remnant glows.

The Belmont Prairie Nature Preserve is a wedge of about ten acres of tallgrass tucked into an unlikely spot between a golf course, freeways, and subdivisions, deep in the Chicago suburbs. Look west across the prairie and you can't help but think of a more subdued Albert Bierstadt painting in the Hudson River School style, or perhaps the shadowy drama of an Andrew Wyeth rural landscape.

Turn in another direction, and the view is more "Chicago Suburban School of Realism." Houses. Cars. Roads.

As I walk these and other pockets of remnant prairie in the Chicago suburbs and at Nachusa Grasslands, I marvel at how these tiny prairie acres hung on by a thread when others were destroyed.

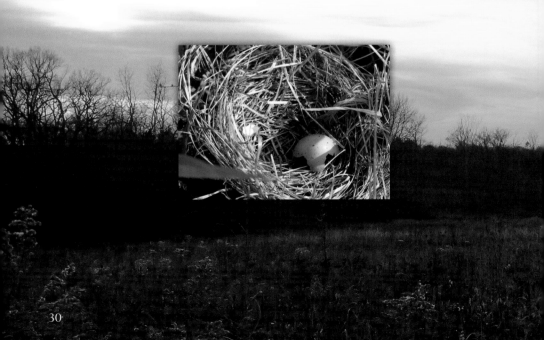

Oh, the stories these plants that remain could tell us! Tales of a time when the Midwest was covered with millions of acres of tallgrass prairie. Survival despite the odds. Most prairie remnant stories revolve around a person who recognized the value of a rare plant, bird, or butterfly and called it to someone's attention before the remnant was bulldozed or developed. I've seen remnants on rocky hills, remnants behind cement plants, remnants in cemeteries. Unexpected islands of original prairie.

So much of what was once here is lost. Gone forever, never to be replaced.

Although only a few thousand of those original acres remain, the ink has not completely faded from the original prairie pages. We read what we see there. Inspired, we continue to plant and reconstruct new prairies for the future.

No matter how many new acres of tallgrass we plant, we can't seem to replicate the original remnants. To come close will require genius, research, and ingenuity—know-how that we don't have yet. And even so, our efforts may not be enough. The planted prairies we create are similar, yet not the same. They are missing some of the necessary insects. Some of the "words" from the original prairie pages. They fail to completely function as the original remnants once did.

If you walk a remnant prairie at sunset, do you feel a different sense of place there than you feel when you walk a planted prairie or a recon-structed prairie? And do you wonder . . . can we ever replicate that?

Perhaps this is not a question any scientist would care to tackle.

We do know this: The remnants we cherish may be the last of their kind. Irreplaceable.

And so, they are almost dreamlike in their tenuous grasp on the land . . . and in their hold on our imagination.

That's why I hike the trails of these prairies. To think about what was lost. To feel that irreplaceable sense of place. To treasure what is left.

And to remember.

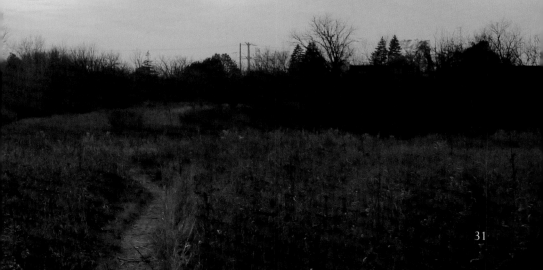

*Thomas Dean*

$A$s I saunter the fourteen acres of Rochester Cemetery in Cedar County, Iowa, on Memorial Day, I traverse the ground of loss and hope. I'm here mostly to enjoy a notable prairie remnant and native oak savanna, to appreciate the persistence of this chunk of indigenous landscape. I have no relatives buried here, yet the fact that this is also a resting ground for lives lost since the 1830s cannot help but weigh on me.

None of us gets over the loss of loved ones, but we adapt, despite the emptiness in us. When we are at our best, we somehow make our or others' lives better within the circumstances of such loss. I don't know how the human lives remembered here at Rochester Cemetery were lost, though as I walk past the blooming spiderwort and rising bluestem on this Memorial Day, small flags planted in the ground tell me that some certainly suffered death at the hands of war. As I read on the stone monuments names of strangers both long and recently passed, I sense this is a place where grief has been lived and overcome, to the extent we can in a world of loss. And while I gather some measure of peace and hope from the burgeoning spring wildflowers and grasses—the reemergence of prairie life that has continuously survived in this patch of ground for thousands of years—they also remind me of the devastating loss of the native prairie and our need to grieve it.

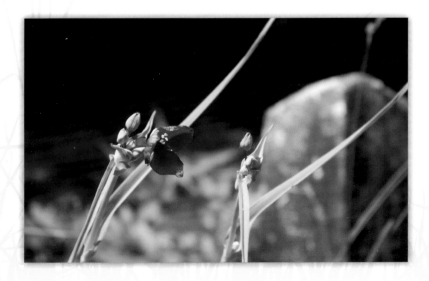

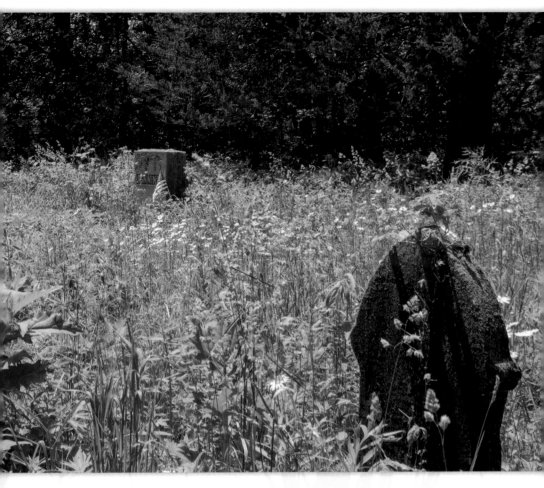

Environmentalists—from scientists to activists to artists—are now calling on us to grieve our losses due to human-caused degradation and destruction of the natural world. We must confront the reality that climate destabilization and other environmental calamities have already caused great losses and will continue to do so. A recent study published by the National Academy of Sciences reported that since the rise of human civilization, half of the planet's plants and 83 percent of its wild mammals have disappeared. By another measure, half of the planet's wildlife has vanished since I was a teenager in the 1970s. Everyone knows that to recover from the loss of our loved ones, we must grieve. If we are to have any hope of relieving the anguish of solastalgia—a neologism for the distress wrought by environmental change—and of moving toward a positive future for our planet, we must acknowledge and grieve our massive losses.

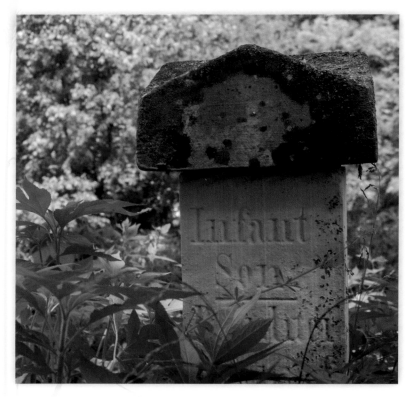

Grief is not hopelessness. It can seem like it in the moment, but it is essential to moving forward, to making the best world amidst loss. The tallgrass prairie, in its near-total destruction, is perhaps the greatest environmental loss in human history, and it deserves our grief. But in knowing, acknowledging, and *feeling* what we have lost, the future of prairie can be so much brighter than despair. We know what is gone, and we know we cannot get it back. But our efforts at preservation and conservation of what remains, and at reconstruction and restoration of some of what we've lost, can make of this wounded world a much better place.

On that Memorial Day in Rochester Cemetery, grief, honored remembrance, and love of the prairie—and I believe hope for its future—coalesced for me. Such moments are welcome in the wake of loss and the crucible of hope.

# HEALING

*Cindy Crosby*

*A*hhhhh—chooo! *Echinacea.* The name almost sounds like a sneeze, doesn't it?

So perhaps it's not surprising that the pale purple coneflower of the Midwestern prairie, *Echinacea pallida*, is used for medicine. Specifically, for fighting colds.

Two other species used medicinally are purple coneflower (*Echinacea purpurea*) and narrow-leaved purple coneflower or "black Samson" (*Echinacea angustifolia*). Even though it isn't native to my county in Illinois, I have the purple coneflower in my backyard garden. Pretty! The goldfinches love the seeds.

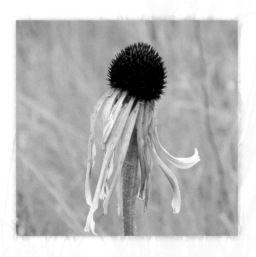

When I teach prairie ethnobotany, my students love to hear how some Native Americans smeared the juice of coneflowers on their hands. They then plunged their hands painlessly into boiling water or were able to handle hot items without flinching. Hurts just to think about it, doesn't it?

This pretty plant was, for its time, a botanical trip to the pharmacy. When chewed, the coneflower root helped numb toothache pain. Coneflowers were also made into concoctions used as a remedy for sore throats and as an antidote for snakebite.

The scientific name for pale purple coneflower comes from the Greek, *echinos*, meaning "sea urchin" or "hedgehog." Take a look at the spiky center. Appropriate, isn't it?

The Mayo Clinic notes that *Echinacea* sales make up to 10 percent of the dietary supplement market but offers cautions as to results. There might be better cold remedies today than this prairie icon.

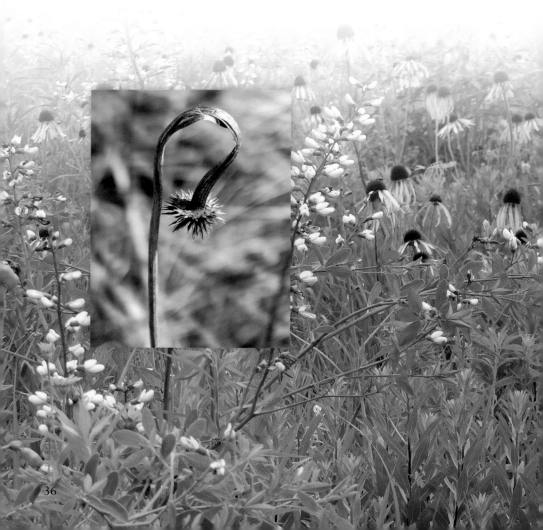

Maybe the best use of pale purple coneflowers is as eye candy on days when the world seems like it is lacking in beauty. Or perhaps the cone-flower's best use is as medicine for the soul.

As the poet Rainer Maria Rilke wrote:

*But because just being here matters, because*
*the things of this world, these passing things,*
*seem to need us, to put themselves in our care*
*somehow. Us, the most passsing of all.*

Feel your spirits lift just looking at them? Me too. Against a backdrop of white wild indigo and bright blue spiderwort, could anything else be prettier? And yet . . . we could lose them all unless we continue to care for our prairies. They need us. And we need them.

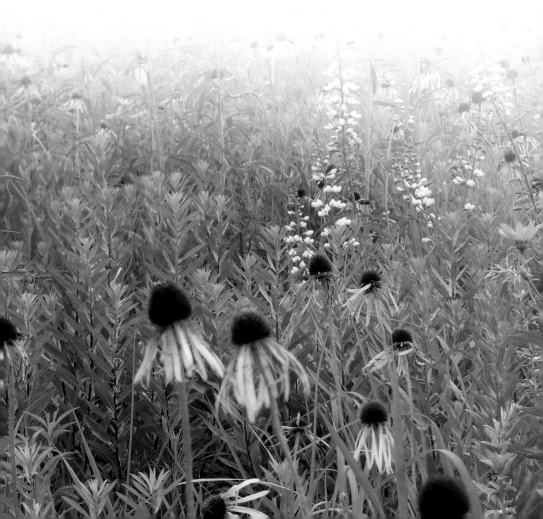

*Thomas Dean*

Wendell Berry in his essay "Health Is Membership" observes that the word "health" derives from the same Indo-European root as "heal," "whole," and "holy." "To be healthy is literally to be whole; to heal is to make whole." Berry says that wholeness arises from "the sense of belonging to others and to our place; it is an unconscious awareness of community, of having in common. . . . The community—in the fullest sense: a place and all its creatures—is the smallest unit of health."

As we seek to heal the prairie, we strive to restore the wholeness of its ecosystem. That's probably not a radical idea to any contemporary conservationist, preservationist, or restorationist. Yet when we heal the prairie, we also heal ourselves—we make ourselves more whole—by widening our sense of belonging to the community, in Berry's (and Aldo Leopold's before him) fullest definition. Prairie becomes not just a familiar landscape but the model of our own health.

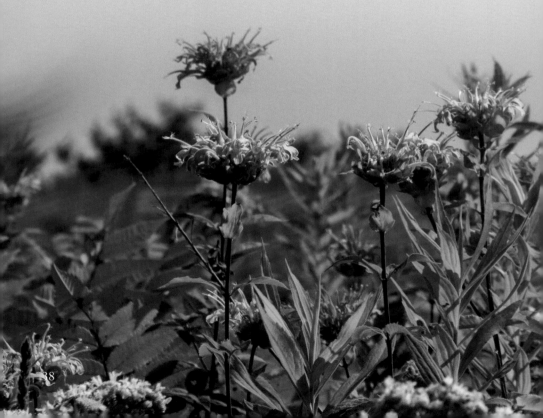

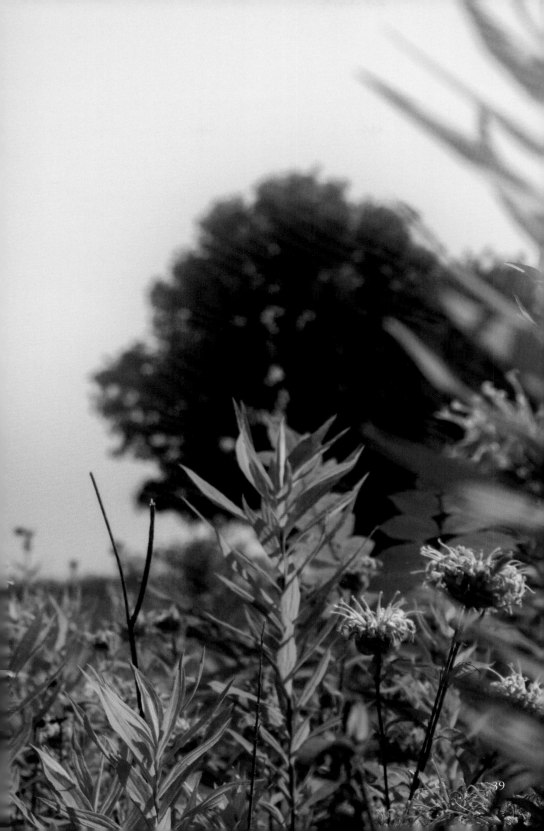

Berry was not talking specifically about the prairie in his essay, or about any particular type of land. Berry's "the land" is a whole place—the whole of the earth. The prairie, then, is a member of the community that includes forests, deserts, oceans—everything. When one member of the community is ill, all are ill. Bringing one member of the community back to health contributes to the health of the whole. So when we work to bring the bergamot, Culver's root, and rattlesnake master (all with medicinal qualities, by the way) back to full bloom in our local prairie, we are not only healing our local land; we are also in part helping to bring back the blue whale from the brink of extinction. And in so doing, we are also making ourselves whole beings again.

Wendell Berry writes from a Christian perspective, but even the atheists amongst us may acknowledge this as "holy" work, given the etymological relationships with health and wholeness. As Berry says, "I don't think mortal healers should be credited with the power to make holy. But I have no doubt that such healers are properly obliged to acknowledge and respect the holiness embodied in all creatures." Heal–health–whole–holy. It is all one. We are all one.

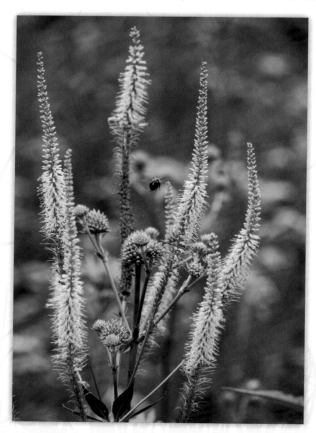

# REMNANT

*Thomas Dean*

*I* am a collector of remnants. In remnants, I find reality and authenticity. Among my prized possessions are a discarded roofing shingle from Sigurd Olson's Listening Point cabin and a bundle of red pine bark shavings I debarked, as part of a Land Ethic Leader service project, from a "Leopold tree"—a tree that Aldo Leopold family members had planted decades ago on the land at the Shack in Wisconsin. When the gold-topped dome of the University of Iowa's 1840 Old Capitol (the first state capitol building) burned in a construction accident, the next day I scoured the ash-laden grounds for a few charred remnants, which now sit on my office desk in the building next door.

Sigurd Olson's Listening Point cabin has a new roof. Many Leopold trees have been repurposed into a beautiful green Leopold Foundation building. The UI's Old Capitol has a shiny rebuilt dome sitting proudly atop

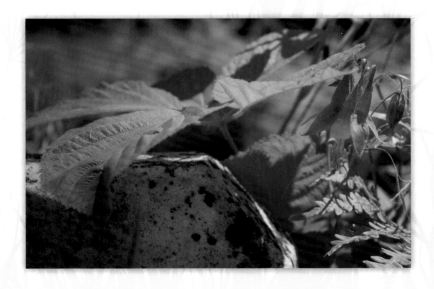

the historic building. While all these projects had preservation at their heart, loss—loss, in part, of authenticity and reality—has been inevitable. Such irretrievable loss is why I am compelled to gather remnants, to hold authenticity. Remnants are a stay against loss.

I truly love to enter the grandeur of endless tallgrass at Iowa's Neal Smith Wildlife Refuge, one of the largest prairie restorations in the country, or any number of smaller reconstructed prairies. But the most authentic prairie experience possible is not in restorations, which by definition have lost their direct lineage to a continuous ecosystem, but in remnants, where native plants are the discarded original elders of the tallgrass. Ironically, remnants are usually where human intervention is flagrant, if not pervasive: hillsides among farm fields, cemeteries, ditches along railbeds and roads. Prairie remnants often exist because they are "worthless," pieces of native land on the margins that cannot be turned to utility or profit.

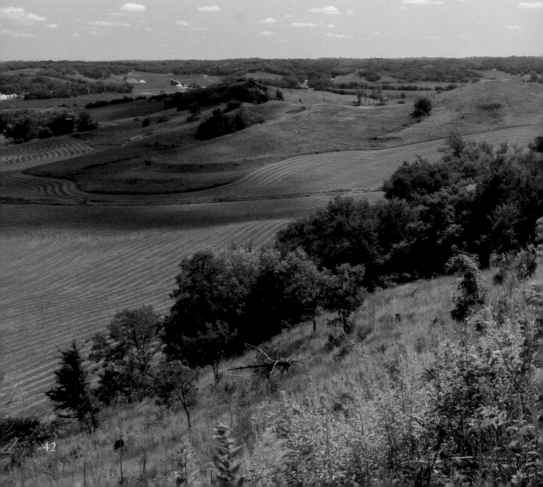

Fortunately, some prairie stewards choose to care for these indigenous authentics, the most "real" of the 0.1 percent of prairie acreage that remains in Iowa. Far to the west of my home in Iowa City, I can feel, smell, and touch the original prairie on Hitchcock Nature Center's Badger Ridge in the Loess Hills above the farm fields that spread out below me. A few miles to the east of my home, I can walk among Rochester Cemetery's truly native spiderwort and columbine that embrace the stone monuments on the graves of the fallen.

Of course, I control my fingers that itch to acquire the authentic, to take with me a totem of the original tallgrass. I leave the ancient bee balm and milkweed pods behind so as not to break the primeval cycle still emerging from these small places. On the prairie, the remnant is original renewal, not inventive replication. It is the remains of the real in a world of artifice.

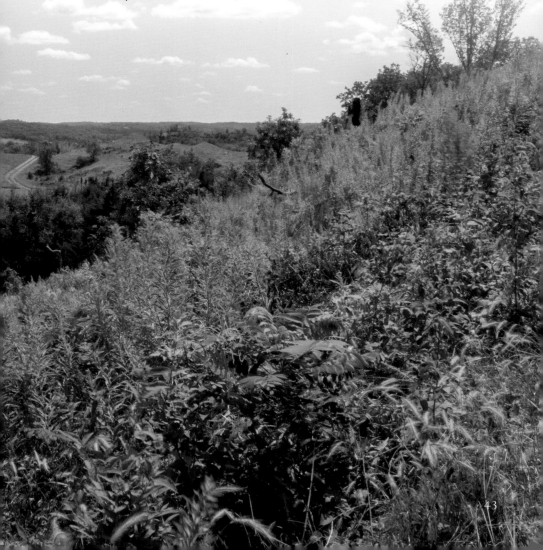

## Cindy Crosby

Dr. Gerould Wilhelm is in the house. My house, in fact. Talking about prairie remnants.

When I moved to the Chicago suburbs twenty years ago, I was despondent over the home we purchased in a busy suburban subdivision. Tiny plots of land. Cookie-cutter houses. But . . . good schools. Easy access to my husband's new job. Those were trade-offs—all good things!—but they didn't salve my need for "nature," which I believed at the time was anywhere but here.

Then I met my backyard neighbor.

I was planting a little prairie strip by our shed with the native plants I was newly learning to love as part of my own transplant process to Illinois. Putting down roots in both a literal and physical sense. Dr. Wilhelm stood in his yard, which was devoid of lawn and bursting with (I would soon learn) more than three hundred species of plants. A few neighbors had complained to me about it. Too lazy to mow!

Jerry took one look at my prairie patch. A big smile crossed his face. "Bless your heart!" Offers of plant plugs and advice soon followed. My neighbor was, as it turned out, an eminent taxonomist. His *Plants of the Chicago Region* and later his ten-pound book, *Flora of the Chicago Region*, would become my bibles as a naturalist and prairie steward.

Almost two decades after this encounter, I invited him to talk to a group of naturalists over dinner at our house about his life's work. More than forty

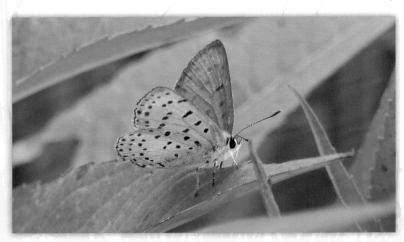

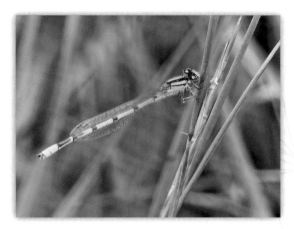

people eagerly soaked up his words. I've forgotten much of what he said, but what stuck with me was this: our prairie remnants are irreplaceable.

In Illinois, where once at least twenty-two million acres of tallgrass covered the state, less than twenty-three hundred acres of high-quality remnant prairie remain. Much of this original prairie is being recreated as "planted prairies" by restorationists like myself, who try to replicate what was lost. As a steward for a one-hundred-acre planted prairie, I appreciate what this prairie reconstruction does to help pollinators recover and to show people the beauty of the original tallgrass.

But when I walk through a prairie remnant—that original piece of tallgrass that somehow escaped the plow—I feel a tingling in my soul. It's difficult to put my finger on the difference. But there is a sense of the past, of something special, that just doesn't happen in a planted prairie.

All feelings aside, I appreciate the science behind preserving these remnants. What Dr. Wilhelm teaches us is that the original prairie, encapsulated in these remaining tracts, is irreplaceable. These remnants are their own world, one that we have not learned to replicate. We can turn old agricultural fields into prairie, but we can't completely replace what was lost. Not yet.

Which means these remnants that remain—these precious prairie remnants—must never be traded for development or tamed for those who demand a more orderly, groomed look. Along the roadsides and railroad tracks, in the corners of old farm fields. In cemeteries or on top of rocky knobs. We must guard those little worlds at all costs.

In a world of throwaway, replaceable convenience items and instant gratification, these few remaining prairie remnants hold secrets we don't understand. Keys to the history of our land that we call home in the Midwest. The soil. The insects. The plants. Everything in a remnant interacts in a way we haven't been able to replicate.

It's up to us to take care of what remains.

*conversation eight*

# RESTORATION

*Cindy Crosby*

The Greek word *apokathístēmi* means to "restore back to its original standing." Whenever the science of prairie restoration seems like Greek to me, I remind myself that prairie restorationists and artists—as well as scientists—also have a lot in common. Although we think of restoration as a science, it's also about creativity.

Prairie restoration begins with a vision. The dream of how the land might be healed, imagined in the mind of a steward or site manager.

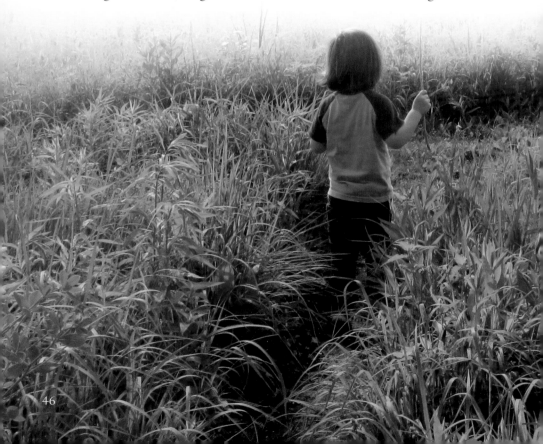

There's a lot of trial and error. Preliminary sketching, if you will; a few rough drafts. Sometimes, you scrap everything—plow the whole prairie planting under—and start over.

There may be misunderstandings along the way. People who don't get it. They look at your "project" and shake their head. They wonder out loud if you have wasted your time. "Weeds. What a mess!" Every prairie volunteer, steward, or site manager has heard that one before. First-time visitors to the prairie have thought it. And who can blame them? It's difficult to understand what you haven't taken time to get to know. Prairies take an investment of time. You remind yourself of this. As a restorationist, you keep on moving forward. You believe in what you are doing. You look for the breakthroughs.

Restore. "To bring back." This assumes something precious was lost. Something worth the time, energy, and thought to replace. The definition continues, "to its original health or vigor." Not just reviving the land. Seeing it completely repaired. No small thing.

Almost all of the original tallgrass prairie has vanished. Lost to the plow, to development, and to perhaps, a lack of imagination. Most of the prairie restorations you see today are actually replanted prairies. A few precious thousands of acres are the original remnant tallgrass prairie.

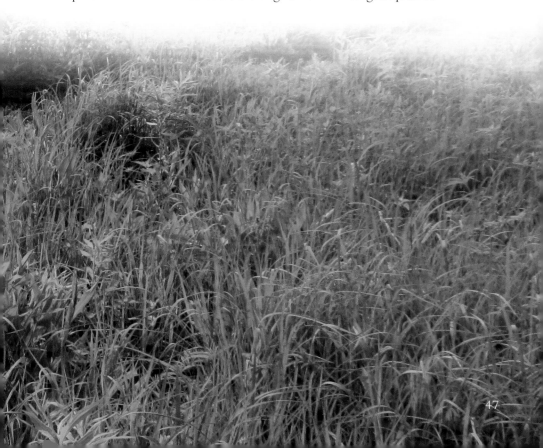

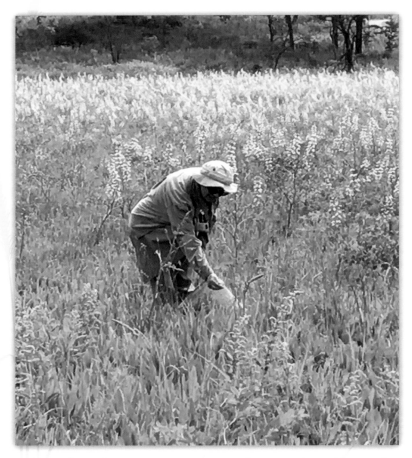

From these ghosts, we try to recreate what once was and learn what we have lost. We see the relationships that exist there and try to replicate them. We learn that no matter how much we try, it's impossible to quite make our plantings the same. But still, we strive for that impossible goal.

Without imagination—without creativity—without courage—the best prairie restorations don't happen. The rewards don't always come in our lifetime. But the work we do isn't for ourselves, although the tallgrass is gratifying in a thousand different ways. We work, knowing we leave a legacy for those who will come after us. We think of them as we drip with sweat, freeze, or pull weeds . . . plant seeds.

There is an art to restoring a prairie. We can see the future tallgrass community in our minds. Envision it. *That end result*. And as all prairie lovers and restorationists know, it's worth the creative effort. Worth the work.

Worth the wait.

## Thomas Dean

*I* can't believe I'm standing in the middle of the world's second ecological restoration—at the Leopold Shack near Baraboo, Wisconsin. And I can't believe I'm pulling out native plants from this historic ground.

In 1935, Aldo Leopold (born and raised on the banks of the Mississippi in Burlington, Iowa) and his family began a historic effort on a worn-out farm he had purchased along the Wisconsin River. The previous year, Aldo and his colleagues had spearheaded the *first* ecological restoration in the world, the University of Wisconsin Arboretum in Madison, which includes the Curtis Prairie. Transporting this radical idea onto his nearby private land, Leopold and family lovingly turned the abandoned chicken coop into the now-legendary Shack and began replanting a mixed woods and prairie landscape devastated by ignorance.

Today, the restored prairie at the Shack thrives, but it must be managed. Leopold himself rarely used the word "restoration," being more likely to say

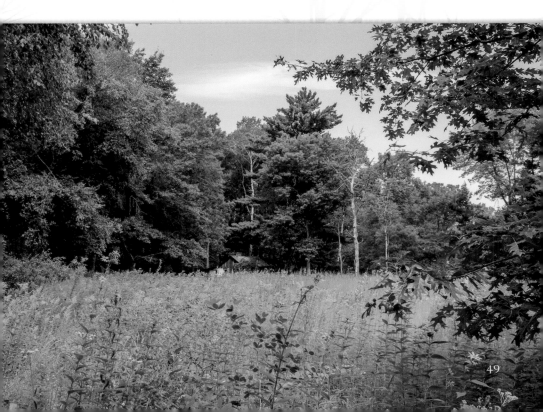

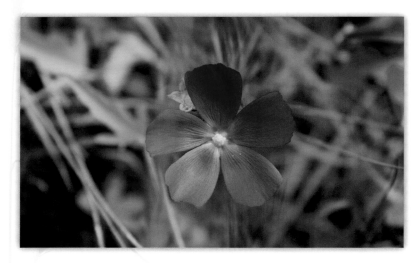

he was "healing the wounded land." The healing of a human wound does not return the body precisely to its original state. Likewise, once disturbed, land cannot really be returned exactly to its previous condition. Opportunistic native plants, not just invasive species, can challenge prairie restoration. Goldenrod is native to the tallgrass prairie but also aggressive. Leave it alone and your diverse prairie could become colonized by significant stretches of tiny golden late-summer flowers.

Part of my training as a Land Ethic Leader through the Aldo Leopold Foundation included a service project. One of our tasks was to cull goldenrod from the prairie at the Shack. So indeed here I was, pulling native plants out of the second ecological restoration in the world! I was treading the same ground where Aldo and family had spent years planting, managing, and replanting in this historic prairie. Although my labor was brief and my effort small in scope, as I tugged the colonizing stalks from the sandy Wisconsin soil, amazement at the historic continuum I found myself within flooded my awareness.

My visits to the Shack and the Leopold Center a half-mile down the road have always been significant restorative events for me. Whether I am participating in a writing workshop with Kim Blaeser at the Shack, attending the dedication of the new memorial at the site of Aldo's death with his daughter Estella sharing words with us, enjoying a Scott Russell Sanders reading or conference reception at the gorgeous center building, or just sauntering along the woodland path to the Leopold Great Marsh, my spirit and my faith in the land ethic are always restored. But I have yet to quite replicate the restorative inspiration of standing amidst the swaying grasses and forbs of the prairie at the Shack on a beautiful breezy September day, placing my hand to the soil worked by Aldo Leopold himself, and contributing a few moments to the healing of this very special wounded land the great conservationist had envisioned and practiced so many decades ago.

# LISTENING

*Cindy Crosby*

Waves of sandhill cranes scribble their way across the sky in early March. It's a choreography of sorts, an aerial ballet. Weirdly prehistoric. On the ground, these ungainly birds—four feet high, with wingspans that may reach seven feet across—look gawky. Yet in the air, they take on energy and grace that stops my breath.

They are not holding their breath, however. The vocal cords of the sandhill cranes were said by John James Audubon to stretch to five feet. He noted that their calls may reverberate for three miles. No wonder their eerie cries echo through my house, even with the windows closed! Over the mashed-down tallgrass of the late winter prairie where I stand, the wide-open sky is full of their racket.

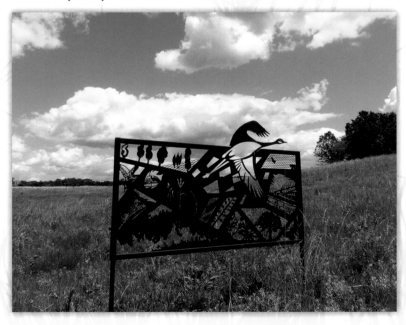

Every spring, the sandhill cranes make their way north across the Chicago suburbs. The cranes are moved by some inner compulsion, some signal that tells them go, Go, GO! Unlike the Canada geese, which now short-stop in our area all winter, the cranes do not fly in a straight "V." Rather, they move determinedly in that formation for a bit, then pause. Suddenly, they swirl and turn, like the writing of a calligrapher who has had too much caffeine and lost control of her pen. To some on the ground, it may look like confusion or chaos. But to me, it is all joyful dance.

Today, I hike the Schulenberg Prairie at the Morton Arboretum in Lisle, Illinois, the first prairie I ever understood as such when I moved to the Chicago suburbs. At one hundred acres, it is a middling-sized prairie, not nearly as large as some (Midewin National Tallgrass Prairie to the south will be more than twenty thousand acres), but much bigger than the prairie patch I have cultivated in my small backyard. The sweep of blue over the Schulenberg offers virtual paper for the skywriting of the cranes.

The first wave of about thirty cranes has passed. There's a pause. The others are not far behind. Waves and waves—hundreds, then thousands—of sandhill cranes.

How do you describe the sandhill crane's song to someone who has never heard it? The first time I listened to their calls, I only knew it was something unusual. Something different. The sound of the sandhill cranes is like a purring cat. It is a thrumming of blood, sporadic, a vibration. If I can hear it from far below on the ground, what must that racket sound like in the swirling tornado of birds?

As I hike, looking up, a sun halo rainbows the sky, creating a backdrop of unending promise. Change, like the migration of the cranes, has its own predictable rhythms: joy, loss, happiness, grief. There is comfort in this. I know the cranes will return in November on their way south. Predictable. But never taken for granted.

I listen and watch for the next wave, shielding my eyes against the sun.

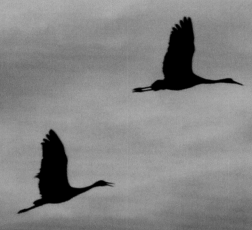

*Thomas Dean*

What does it mean to listen to the prairie?

I hear the chirps, songs, and alarms of goldfinches, meadowlarks, and red-winged blackbirds. I hear the snaps, whirs, and buzzes of summer insects among the grasses. I hear the breeze sighing through the plant stalks, a gentle swish in summer; a harsher, reedy rustling in fall; a cold, hollow rattle in winter.

I hear all these beautiful sounds, but am I really listening to the prairie? Is listening more than attention to the auditory vibrations resonating in my ears? How else might we "listen," especially in an age when human attitudes and activities are so harmful to the natural world?

Listening to nature is much more profound than trading mere words, if that were even possible. When we observe the natural world closely, we depend on intuition, feeling, and sensing to know what it is "saying." When we notice the proliferation of invasive plant species, or even opportunistic natives, the prairie is telling us that the ground remains disturbed and

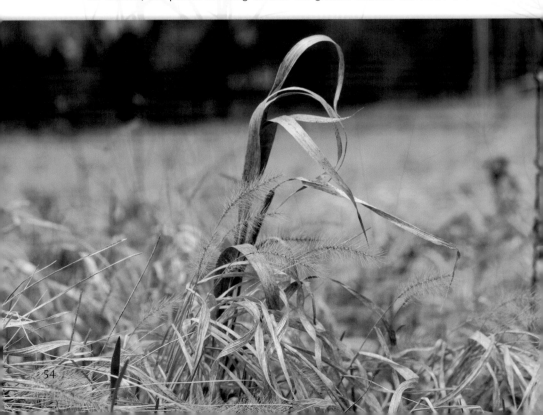

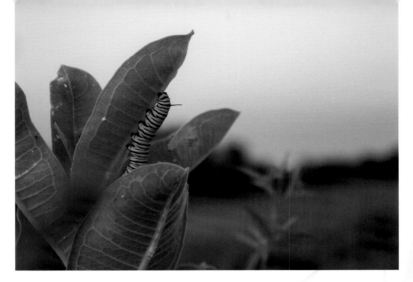

continues to need human intervention and care. When the song of the meadowlark and bobolink go silent, the prairie is lamenting the loss of its extent that has provided habitat for these winged migrants. When the diversity of the prairie flora unfolds in its summer glory, it tells us, "Our strength, our life, is in interdependence, as should be yours." When the first sign of green emerges from the prairie soil in early spring, the prairie tells us, "Your trust in nature is well placed."

Perhaps the greatest difficulty in listening to the prairie—or any part of nature—is that we must come in humility, even vulnerability. Writer Belden Lane says, "Communication in its deepest form is always rooted in a shared vulnerability, a mutual convergence of vulnerabilities." Those aren't ideas that most Americans cater to. But to hear both the wisdom and wounds of nature—and to realize we are the perpetrators of those wounds and that we need to be the students of that wisdom—we need to take that very difficult first step in conversation: to listen.

This is not an entirely mystical or "New Age" idea. Listening to plants is what earned cytogeneticist Barbara McClintock a Nobel Prize in Physiology or Medicine in 1983. As Linda Hogan says in *Dwellings: A Spiritual History of the Living World* regarding McClintock's work on gene transposition in corn plants, "Her method was to listen to what corn had to say, to translate what the plants spoke into a human tongue." McClintock "came to know each plant intimately. She watched the daily green journeys of their growth from earth toward sky and sun. . . . Her approach to her science was alive, intuitive, and humane. . . . She saw an alive world, a fire of life inside plants." McClintock herself said that we must "hear what the material has to say to you. One must have a feeling for the organism."

The more profoundly we listen to nature, the more we are open to the teachings we need from it and the more we comprehend its needs from us. As long as there is prairie—native, remnant, or restoration—it is speaking profoundly to us about our relationship with it. It is our obligation—and our honor—to listen.

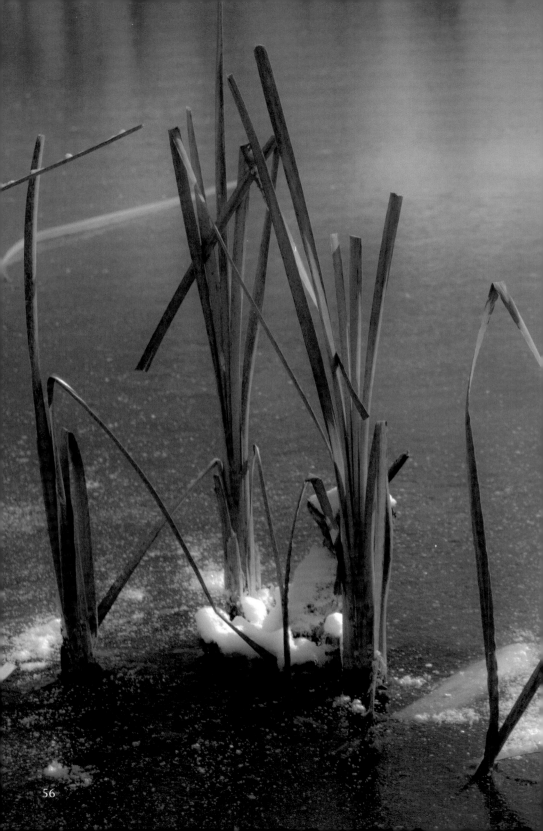

# STILLNESS

*Thomas Dean*

In Wendell Berry's well-known poem, the speaker, in despair and fear over the modern world, retreats to the titular "peace of wild things," where ducks and herons rest and feed. The speaker finds this peace, this grace and freedom, in "the presence of still water."

Close to home, I find the peace of wild things, the stillness that the troubled speaker of Berry's poem seeks, in the prairie. The moment I step onto the path into the grassland, my breathing slows and my mind clears as my eyes take in the sprawling expanse of natural bounty, whether in full bloom or at rest. I admit it requires some deliberate effort, some mindfulness on my part to leave cares behind me. But it doesn't take long for my mental, physical, and emotional focus to sharpen on the wonders surrounding me, and for the pulse of my being to harmonize with the grasses and forbs.

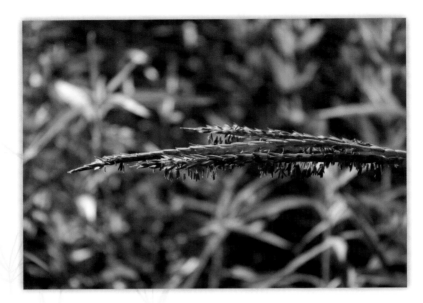

But of course the prairie is hardly "still." I am reminded of that when trying to capture an image in a photo, which is often a challenge since the air is always flowing. The delicate grass blades and flower stems are usually in motion, from a leisurely sway to a perpendicular bend at the command of a harsh squall. Meadowlarks and goldfinches flit from stem to stem in search of succulent Asteraceae seeds. Even in the depths of winter, as I contemplate the frozen waters of a prairie pond, the dormant reeds above the ice waver in the wind, and I know life pulses slowly on beneath the ice.

The "stillness" of the prairie is more akin to the "slowness" of the slow movement, which focuses not just on speed. Something "slow"—whether it be food, or cities, or education—embraces quality and authenticity as much as a more leisurely, calmer pace. Likewise, the stillness of the prairie, just as with Wendell Berry's water of the wood drake and heron, rests in its genuineness, its truth, its essential reality. Time and earth play a broader, slower song on the prairie, and when I join its rhythm, my mind, even my soul, is stilled in its measured grace.

*Cindy Crosby*

Reluctance—thy name is spring! At least this year. We've had one of the coldest Aprils on record in the Chicago region. Much grumbling on the part of the natives. After the stillness of winter, we long for birdsong; for the color and snap and jazz of emergence.

The prairies are burned later than usual this season. They are followed by a dry spell. Growth is here, but in slow motion. May arrives, and there's not much in bloom except the fading pasque flowers, always an early arrival, and a few of the more common violets.

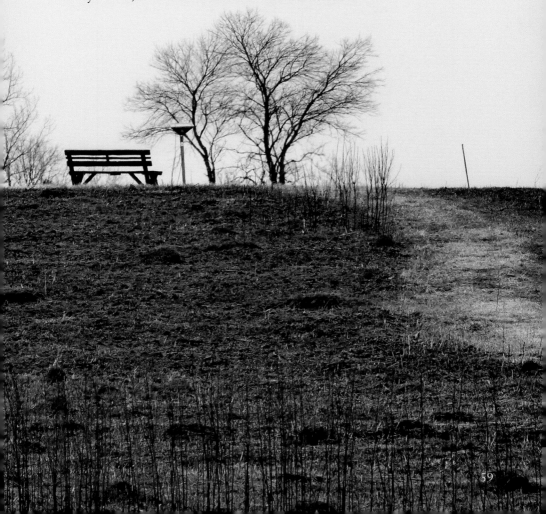

In the prairie savanna the wildflowers are waking up. "Harbinger-of-spring" is blooming, its tiny anthers bright reddish purple. Dutchman's breeches is throwing a party; wild ginger and bluebells hint at blooms on the way. Mayapples are bulleting through the soil and unfolding their umbrellas. Once again, I have to remind myself of the different ways to tell apart the anemones: wood, rue, and false. Spring beauties and bloodroot are in full bloom, and trout lilies glint white and yellow under the trees.

On the prairie, tiny compass plants offer their own delights as miniature versions of their soon-to-be-grown-up selves. Wood betony, known also by its less attractive name of "lousewort," crinkles into bud. Those rhubarb-red leaves! Unmistakable in the dust of the prairie soil. The grasses needle their way into view. The prairie turns a furry green. Mounds of anthills are clearly visible now, and prairie dropseed humps evoke a fleet of UFOs landing.

I find myself responding to the leisurely, more deliberate pace of the prairie by slowing down as well. For the first time in many months, I take my sketch pad out to the prairie and sit with the plants, just observing. There's a buzz and hum of motion; the early pollinators are out and about. Bee flies. Ants. Honeybees. Numerous native bees, so difficult to identify and so important to the life of the prairie.

By July, the tallgrass will be a frenzied rush-hour collision of pollinators, blooms, competing grasses, and birds. Bright colors, all jostling for my attention. So many species! So much glitz and light and sound. My pace will increase as well—so much to see! So much as a steward to do! My attention will be pulled in a thousand different directions.

For now, I'm savoring the stillness. Discovering what the prairie has to teach me in this moment.

Letting this be the pause that energizes for the busy season ahead.

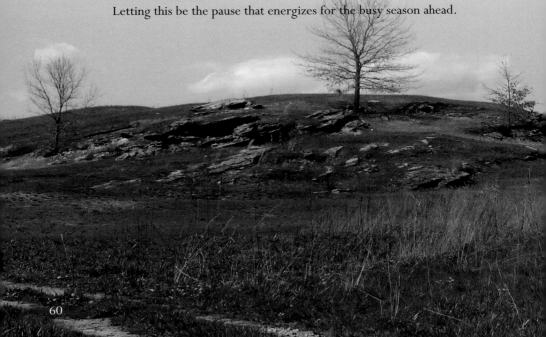

# PATIENCE

## Cindy Crosby

*L*ately it seems I've been invited to practice patience. Sit in hospital waiting rooms. Long hours of car travel. Trains that didn't run as scheduled. Cancelled flights. Jets that sat on the tarmac without taking off. Listening to endless loops of "on hold" music on the phone while watching time tick away. Anxious hours waiting for our granddaughter to be born.

Waiting for a response from someone I emailed weeks ago about a project. Waiting for the temperature to warm up past zero so I can hike longer than twenty minutes at a stretch.

Waiting. Waiting. Waiting.

If I slow down and pay attention to my life, I see particular patterns emerge. Certain messages are repeated. Often, the messages and patterns are all about my need to relearn patience. Take things slowly. Sit with decisions. Wait.

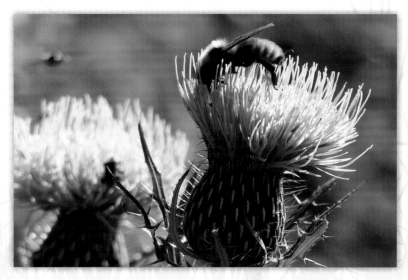

In my mid-fifties, I blew out my knee while hiking in the snow and ice on the 606, Chicago's terrific urban trail. Since then, I've become much more aware of my own limitations. Because I have to physically slow down, it's forced me to slow down in other ways. To become more attentive. More patient with myself. More patient—hopefully—with others. But I can't say it's been easy.

Until I was forced to slow down, I thought I was a pretty patient person. But there's nothing like congratulating yourself on a virtue you think you have to discover how pitiful your abilities really are. *Patience? Let's see what she's got.* You quickly realize your illusions about yourself.

Those of us who love the tallgrass and work with prairie restoration are well acquainted with patience. We know the power of waiting. Nothing worthwhile happens on the prairie without it. Some prairie seeds hang on through the winter, waiting for the optimal time to drop. We weed white sweet clover year after year, trying to knock it back. We mark time after planting the leadplant seeds, which may take several years to

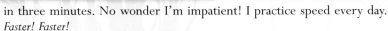

flower. Progress is slow. There is little instant gratification in prairie restoration.

Our world values speed. It values brevity. It promotes instant gratification. I can order groceries with a click of a button; they'll be at my door in an hour. Need a book? In a few minutes, I can download one from my library to my laptop. My microwave can turn a frozen entree into a hot Thai dish in three minutes. No wonder I'm impatient! I practice speed every day. *Faster! Faster!*

The prairie reminds me that many good things take patience. The pale purple coneflowers and stands of big bluestem are echoes of numerous cycles of freeze and fire; sprout and leaf; bud and bloom.

Each spring, the prairie is touched by flame. Floods of flowers follow. None of this can be rushed. It's part of the beauty of the whole. A cycle. And that's what makes it so meaningful.

Try thinking in "prairie time," I remind myself. Slow might be the way to go. Don't be in such a hurry. Take a deep breath. Sit with things for a while. Try not to react by pushing yourself to do more in less time.

Let the prairie be your guide.

*Thomas Dean*

As I drove home from a spring nature photography workshop with Minnesota's Bryan Hansel and John Gregor at the Neal Smith National Wildlife Refuge near Prairie City, Iowa, my camera-obsessed eye could not help but see everything outside my car's window as a picture. In my sight, the principles of perspective, line, shape, pattern, texture, echo, and visual flow and weight tied hills to fields, connected trees to windmills, linked land and sky in layers and tones—linked the "loose parts" of nature into an understanding of the whole.

In *The Nature Principle*, Richard Louv extends to adults his idea of children's "nature deficit disorder"— loss of perceptual skill, creative play, and well-being due to disconnection from the natural world. Louv harks back to architect Simon Nicholson's 1970s idea that working with "loose parts" in our environment—materials that can be moved around, redesigned, taken apart, and put back together without preset directions—can drive and enhance creativity. Louv says, "Exposure to the loose but related parts of nature can encourage a greater sensitivity to patterns that underlie all experience, all matter, and all that matters" and "the ability to see patterns in the universe, to detect hidden links between what is and what could be."

Connecting loose parts takes patience, as does making photos, both having greatly enriched my relationship with prairie. To take a good photo, I must be still and look with purpose and intent. The beauty and patterns among flowers, grasses, rises and swales, clouds, birds, butterflies, even the litter beneath my feet are gradually revealed as I patiently pay deeper and deeper attention. I determine the best camera settings and snap the shutter, and my apperception of the loose parts before me leads to, I hope, an aesthetically pleasing image.

But much more is also happening. Through patience, my immersion in this natural place yields discernment much deeper than what the camera has apprehended. Making a picture is only a doorway, a first step through to the infinite beauty and meaning of the living world.

After the shutter snaps, the colors and tones of shooting star and blue sky deepen further for me. The lines of last year's bluestem and still-bare oak branches in the distant savanna extend infinitely beyond my sight. Visual echoes of horizon line and prairie burn's edge redound, and audible echoes of wind brushing last year's brittle grasses merge with meadowlark song. I smell the softening topsoil, connecting me to the deep roots quickening below. All my senses open, and the interdependent web of the biotic community invites me to acknowledge my own living presence, right here and now.

Yes, I get all that from taking a picture. I could never have this experience of the living world from only a screen, even a camera's LCD screen, despite their millions of bits, bytes, and megapixels. Taking nature photographs calls for my patience and focuses my attention so I may begin to perceive and connect the endless loose parts of the natural world—the real world.

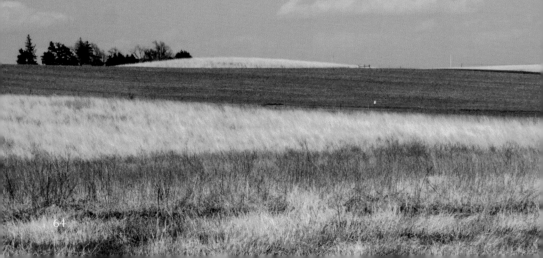

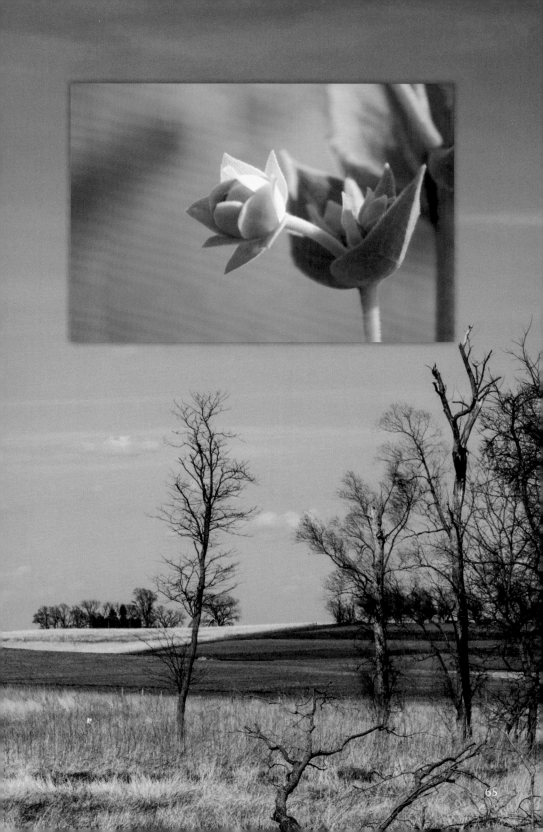

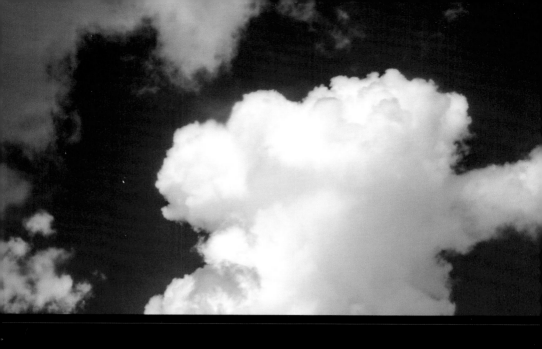

# the spirit of
# CELEBRATION

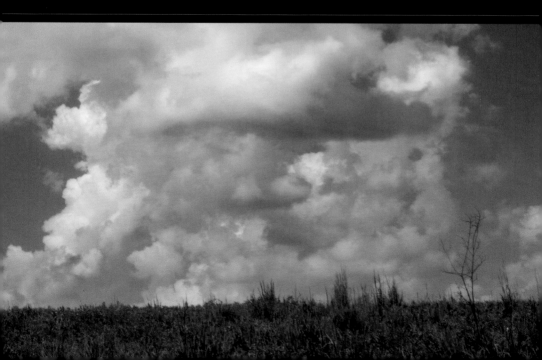

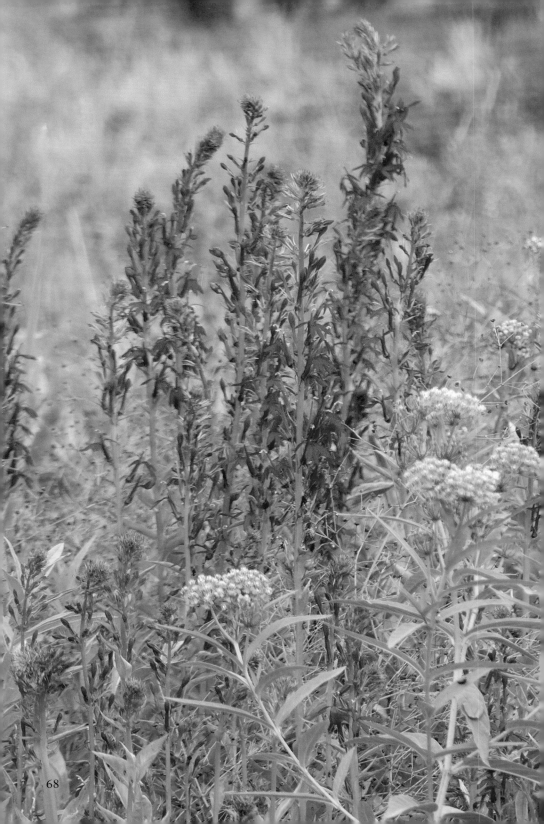

# J O Y

*Cindy Crosby*

*C*ardinal rules on the prairie in early August . . . that is, cardinal flower. Suddenly, she mysteriously appears in the wetlands. Pops up beside the ponds. Strikes scarlet poses throughout the wet prairie.

Her raceme of racy red is unmistakable.

Swallowtail butterflies flock to her. The hummingbirds approve. In my backyard prairie patch and pond they hover, drawn to that screaming scarlet. *Come closer,* the red flowers seem to say. *Wait until you see how sweet we taste.*

Read the field guide descriptions. *Showy.* There's talk about her corollas; those lips! *Juicy. Moist-loving.* Look again. You can't not think of a tube of bright red lipstick, maybe a midlife crisis sports car. This is a sensual flower, make no mistake about it.

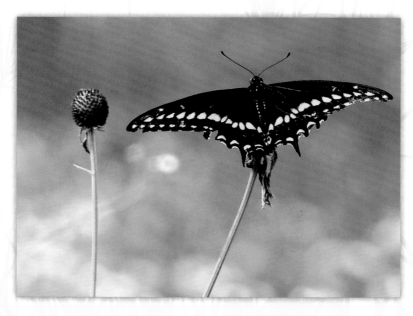

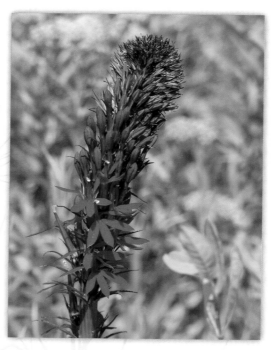

Read on. This plant is "temperamental." Her ecological value to wild-life is categorized as low. But really, who would expect something so ravishing to be useful as well as beautiful?

Although . . . some Native American tribes found cardinal flower roots and blooms important in the making of love charms. The ground-up roots were slipped into food to end arguments and as an antidivorce remedy. Fitting, perhaps, for a bloom so striking to have these supposed powers.

The prairie is not prodigious with its reds. Sure, there is a little royal catchfly sprinkled around. But not a whole lot else that is scarlet.

Purples? Oh my, all over the place! From spring to fall. White—plenty of it. Yellows? The prairie seems to always have something yellow going on. Blue has a voice in some of the springtime savanna flowers and the blue-purples of spiderwort on the prairie. A little blue lobelia in the wetlands. Pinks? Yup. Even pink with a little orange thrown in for good measure.

But red . . . now, that's special.

In my backyard wet prairie, the cardinal flower is elusive. Some years it blooms. Others, it disappears, and I wonder. Is it gone for good? This August—just as I gave up—a few bright red spikes appeared around the prairie pond. I breathed a sigh of relief.

Because what would August be without those splashes of scarlet?

Such joy.

The joy of seeing red.

*Thomas Dean*

One of my greatest joys in life is going to the opera. When the fire curtain goes up at the Lyric in Chicago's Civic Opera House or the maroon curtain rises at the Paramount Theater in Cedar Rapids, I enter a world of transcendent concord. Opera is the grandest art, in which music, story, drama, visual art, and dance cohere in a performance unlike anything else springing from the human imagination. When done well, this integration of art forms immerses me in joy.

On the prairie during a late-summer evening, I hear the distinctive, exuberant "Per-chick-o-ree! Per-chick-o-ree-ree-ree!" of an American goldfinch. My eyes are pulled to the swift undulating flight of the small bird. About twenty feet ahead of me, the olive-hued female alights on the thin stalks of swaying silphium in the warm, slightly humid Iowa evening breeze. I approach as quietly as I can, but the tiny *Spinus tristis* flits away, in search of seeds among the full-blooming prairie plants. She lands skillfully on another nearby delicate stem.

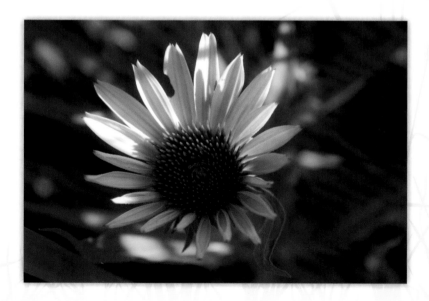

The goldfinch is the prairie's complete avian artist. Its feeding dance is utterly acrobatic, performed on the thin high wire of stems and shoots as the bird dexterously hangs on the seed heads themselves to indulge its appetite. Its song merges, seamless, with its distinctive flight. As the finch flaps its wings to rise on the air currents, it sings. As it folds those wings to glide in a dipping arc, it falls silent. The repetition of this song and dance creates a masterful performance of lyrical rolling waves that aligns sound and image. Staged on the field of greens and yellows against an azure summer sky, the goldfinch's melodic flight and repose are the apotheosis of the art of the prairie.

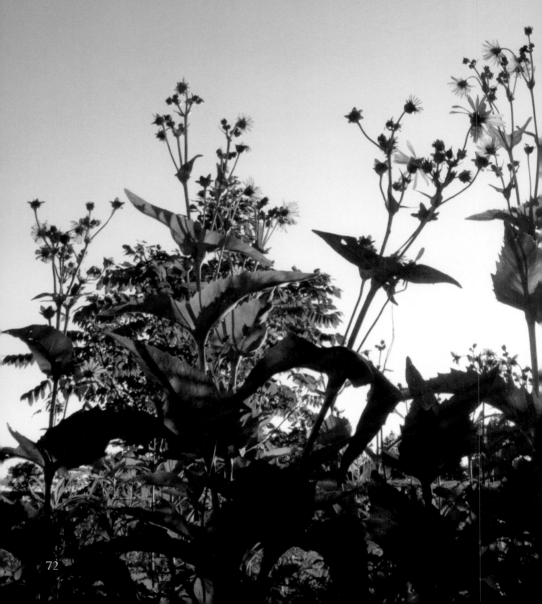

The American goldfinch does not climb to the pinnacle of a high C or tunnel into the chasm of verismo's pathos. It does not bring to life the heights of Tristan and Isolde's sublime bliss or the depths of Pagliaccio's murderous revenge. But its boisterous aria coalesces with its bravura ballet of *grand jeté* flight and *en pointe* feasting here on a gorgeous summer evening on the prairie, bringing me a joy that resembles—and surpasses—the artifice of the opera stage. My joy in the opera is derived from its genius but, admittedly, its human contrivance. My joy in the prairie goldfinch rises from its *genius loci*, the spirit and beauty of nature that no one could possibly replicate on a stage.

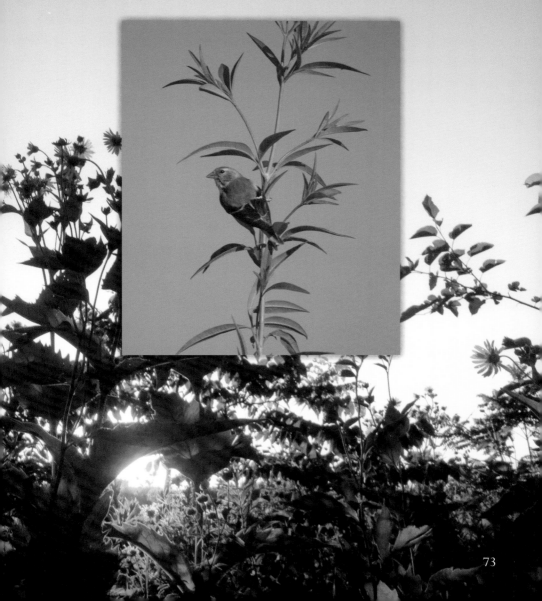

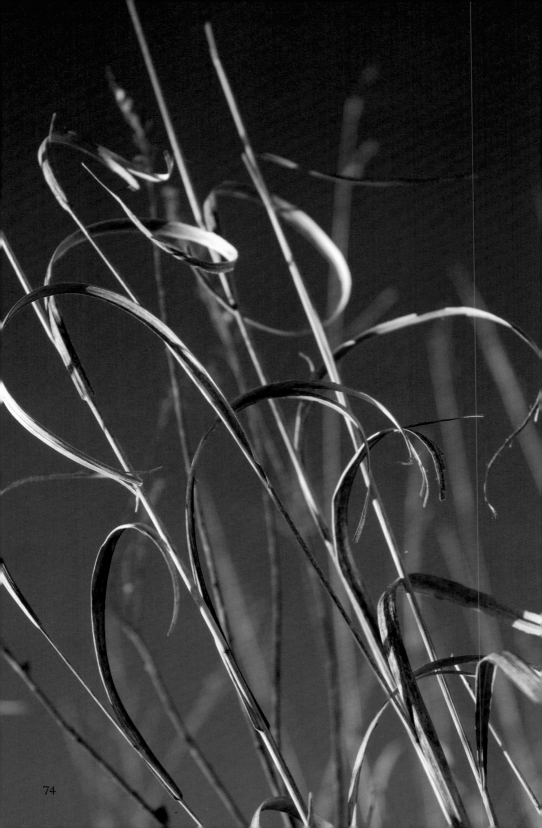

# SURPRISE

*Thomas Dean*

O n a winter day on the prairie, I lie down amidst the dry, dormant stems of tallgrass. Not an activity, I suspect, that would jump to mind for most on a cold February day in Iowa. But new perspective requires bold (well, unusual) action.

As my back crunches down on the crisp litterfall, my eyes gaze upward. Above me play the light brown lines and curves of sleeping bluestem, in relief against the gorgeous high-pressure blue sky. The playful twists and curves flutter just slightly in the breeze, dry remnant streamers of the prairie's flags of summer. But in this quiet time, I delight in surprise. The thin ribbons above me look more like party decorations than nature at rest. I see the prairie at play, not asleep. It's not what I expected. I feel I am fully *in* the prairie in its joyful round of life, not just on the prairie in a time of death.

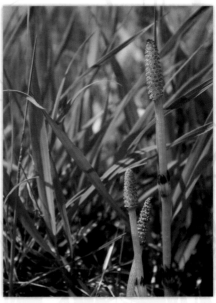

When I visit the prairie, I always try to put expectations aside. Prairie comforts me when I enter its familiarity, but it brings me even greater gifts when I let it surprise me. Sometimes that means looking closer. Sometimes that means listening more intently—both to the song of the prairie itself and the song it raises within me. Sometimes that means putting my whole body among the grasses and forbs in ways I've never experienced before.

I might happen upon a gray tree frog pretending to be invisible on a low broad leaf, having wandered away from the nearby woody area, perhaps in search of a stream. My ears might catch a gentle rustle followed by the tiny, reedy "dick, dick, ciss, ciss, ciss" of a dickcissel foraging on the ground, or the more robust

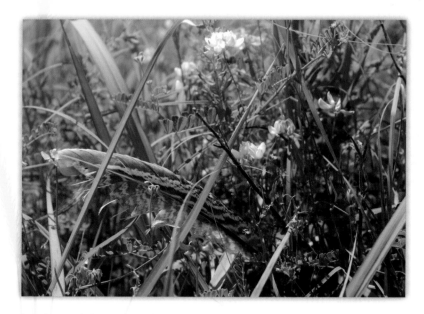

hooting and drumming of a male prairie chicken come a-courting. I might walk past a cluster of bare *Silphium* stems in the brown-gray of winter and marvel at how twisting some can be, in stark dissent from the straight lines of the surrounding grasses. Or I might even stumble across something I've never seen before, such as an emerging horsetail in spring low to the ground, its light tan tubercle-covered cones appearing alien amid the more familiar greening stalks and stems. Or perhaps I might just close my eyes and open my ears, letting the whoosh and whistle of wind, of birdsong, of insect chorus perform its grassland cantata for me.

Whatever the surprise, I let the prairie remind me that it—and the whole natural world—are full of wonders I have yet to experience. Sometimes they cross my path when I least expect it, or perhaps when my mind wanders to the cares of the world beyond this moment, drawing me back to the present in this place. I will experience more surprise with greater intention—by checking my expectations, by changing my perspective, by paying attention.

Look up. Look down. Look inward. Open your eyes. Open your ears. Open all your senses. Open your heart. Look closely. Listen intently. Feel deeply. Let the prairie surprise you . . . so you can see the world anew.

*Cindy Crosby*

Oh, what a difference a little rain makes! Spring has arrived on the prairie—at last!!—in a rush of color and motion. My Tuesday morning volunteer team is updating our plant inventory for our mosaic of prairie, wetlands, and savanna, a task that is into its second season. With the rain comes a flush of new wildflowers. Some familiar. A few surprises.

This spring, we are looking for a hundred or so plants out of the five hundred we believe are here from an inventory more than a decade ago. We looked for them last spring to no avail. We particularly want to find three common but nonetheless elusive plants that we'd missed early in 2017: skunk cabbage, marsh marigold, and rue anemone.

First up is skunk cabbage. Some adventurous members of the team find it barely visible, poking up through the muck in a deep gully. As it matures, the large green leaves make it easier to see. Skunk cabbage is one of the longest-lived wildflowers; writer and naturalist Jack Sanders suggests some specimens may be two hundred years old. Native Americans liked to dry the plant to a fine powder, then use it in tattoos. We check it off our plant inventory, relieved that it's still hanging on at our site.

The marsh marigold—a beautiful, usually somewhat aggressive spring native wildflower—turns out to be a single plant. It is hiding among some fig buttercup (*Ficaria verna*), a pernicious, nonnative invasive wetland species. We'll have to carefully remove the fig buttercup without disturbing the marsh marigold. Left to its own devices, the fig buttercup will take over Willoway Brook, which runs through the prairie.

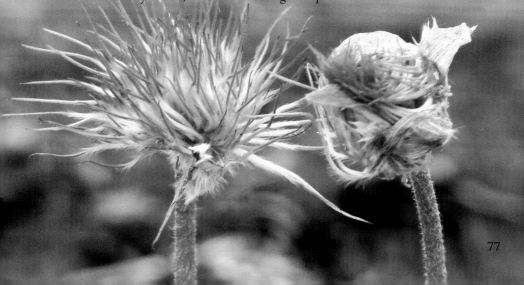

Another missing wildflower, the rue anemone, went from invisible to visible after storms moved through the area and gave everything a shot of grow juice. Such a delicate wildflower, and easy to miss unless you find a large colony. I saw it by accident while gazing at our newly found skunk cabbage. So many amazing things are happening right under our noses! If only we take time to see.

As we looked for the skunk cabbage, marsh marigold, and rue anemone, the plant inventory team found the wildflower harbinger-of-spring for the first time in our savanna. The whole bloom umbel is about the size of my pinkie finger. No wonder we'd missed it!

Most of us are spending our volunteer hours weeding out garlic mustard, a persistent invasive plant that infests disturbed areas around the prairie. As we weed, we discover wild ginger is in bloom. To see the blooms, each leaf must be turned over. You might flip hundreds of wild ginger plant leaves before you find a single flower. The rain also prompted the large-flowered trillium to open, literally overnight. They won't last long. Yellow trout lilies are already going to seed. All around, blooms are throwing themselves into the act of living, dying, and creating more life to follow them before the world heats up.

Spring keeps you on your toes. It reminds you to be amazed. It constantly astonishes you with its sleight of hand. Just when you think you've got a handle on what is blooming, you see something you've never seen on the prairie before. And just when you think you know a flower, it turns up a little different color or gives you a new perspective on its life cycle.

The plant inventory continues. We tally up the numbers, check off plant species, update scientific names that have changed. Enjoy the occasional surprise bloom; mourn the surprising loss of something we thought was common. But no matter how the spreadsheets tally up, we know one thing for certain.

Spring on the prairie was worth the wait.

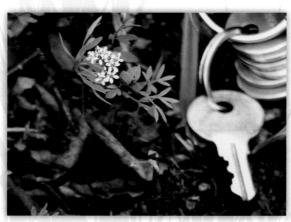

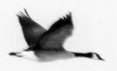

# WONDER

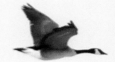

*Cindy Crosby*

Zero. That's the temperature. Not optimal hiking weather on the prairie or for outdoor adventures. But I need the walk. The headlines are full of the latest disasters: earthquakes, school shootings, political unrest. It's easy to slip into despondency.

After more than five decades of wanderings—and at the beginning of a new year—I've been wondering. How do I keep my sense of curiosity and wonder in a cynical world that always seems on the brink of some new disaster?

One of my favorite nature writers, Sigurd Olson, wrote, "While we are born with curiosity and wonder, and our early years full of the adventure they bring, I know such inherent joys are often lost. I also know that, being deep within us, their latent glow can be fanned into flame again by awareness and an open mind."

How do I "fan the flame," "stay aware"? It's so easy to become insular.

Then I look around. Time outdoors. Perhaps that's always the answer.

Even a short walk in the brutal cold is a mental palate cleanser. It sweeps clean the heavy holiday fare. Too much travel. Noise. Not enough time to think.

I breathe in. Exhale. The air sears my lungs, seeps into my gloves, painfully nips my hands. Then all feeling recedes.

Above me, the wild geese fly in formation over the prairie, calling to each other. The sound carries clearly in the cold, crisp air. I inhale again and feel the fuzziness in my mind begin to dissipate.

I think of Mary Oliver's poem "Wild Geese." When I worked as a park ranger on a wilderness island, one of my many unglamorous tasks was sweeping the visitor center floor at the end of the day. As I'd push the broom back and forth, back and forth, I'd try memorizing a new poem each week, written on a card in my pocket. It made the work task more pleasant. "Wild Geese" was one poem that became a favorite.

Lost in remembrance, I almost miss what's under my feet. The prairie and meadow voles have been busy tunneling through the snow on a seed-finding mission. The short winter list of prairie birds and animals is easier to recite than the lengthy roll call of plant species. Winter plant ID is a guessing game. The once-familiar wildflowers have lost their leaves. The grasses are bleached and brittle.

Some I can be fairly certain of, like the thimbleweeds, with their tufts of seeds in various stages of blowout along a sheltered edge of the prairie.

Or the pasture thistle, in its familiar spot next to the path. The compass plant leaf, even when cold-curled like a bass clef, is unmistakable.

But other wildflowers, sans identifying colors, scents, or leaf shapes, are a mystery. Is this one an aster? Sure. But which one? I realize how limited my naturalist skills are every winter.

Such a jumble of seasonal botanical leftovers! All in various stages of decay. Monarda? Check. Blackberry canes? Check. White wild indigo pods? Yup. And is that tiny loop a bit of carrion flower vine? Of course! But which species?

Hours could be spent in this fashion—looking, listening, hypothesizing, thinking, remembering. It takes so little to rekindle the spark of curiosity and wonder. To wake up. To be refreshed.

Just a short hike. A deep breath. A moment's attention toward what's happening around your feet. A glance at the sky.

And suddenly you feel it. The embers of curiosity and wonder begin to glow again.

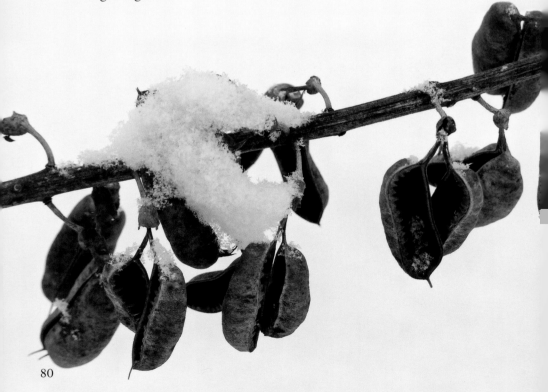

*Thomas Dean*

*T*he shooting star is the wonder of the prairie.

If the prairie had a conscious intent to spark human wonder, the shooting star would be its headliner. One of the first wildflowers to emerge in spring, *Dodecatheon* is simply astonishing. Its blossoming explodes with such exuberance and exquisite beauty, it's hard to believe this is the first gesture of an awakening landscape and not the fireworks of the annual wildflower grand finale.

The complex beauty of a single shooting-star flower, as well as the plant's gorgeous bouquet of endless blooms, entrances me. The elegant corolla of curling white or pink petals bursts open upward, suggesting the points of a star, at the same time they seem to trail away into the ether, mimicking a meteor's tail. The long stamen protruding from the bottom, in bolder yellow and dark red, makes the flower seem to point downward from its nodding cluster, providing the namesake image of a shooting star falling to earth. Few prairie wildflowers have captured the human imagination so robustly.

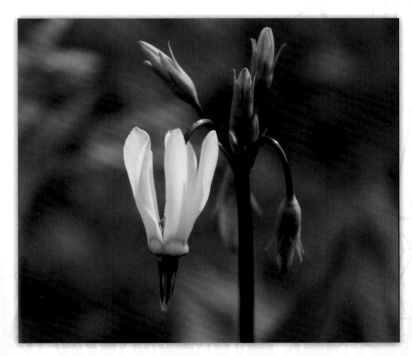

But the shooting star is a prairie ephemeral. It bursts out in brilliant abundance but fades quickly from the spring pantheon, just as a meteor flames magnesium bright and then goes dark in a matter of seconds. The plant is completely dormant by late summer. Another early-season riser, spiderwort, may still put forth a stubborn bloom or two in late July or even August if you're lucky, but the dazzling life of shooting star has been long extinguished, only adding to its wonder.

Rachel Carson in her remarkable long essay *The Sense of Wonder* said, "A child's world is fresh and new and beautiful, full of wonder and excitement." She laments how adulthood dims "that clear-eyed vision, that true instinct for what is beautiful and awe-inspiring." Carson wishes for each child in the world to have "a sense of wonder so indestructible that it would last throughout life." And that sense of wonder for her lies squarely in our need to "turn again to the earth and in the contemplation of her beauties to know the sense of wonder and humility." Carson's prescription is for adults to be companions with children in sharing the "inborn sense of wonder," which also allows the adult to "rediscover . . . the joy, excitement, and mystery of the world we live in." I can think of few prairie plants that would render this joy and wonder better than the shooting star.

I admit that had I found some shooting star as a young boy, my sense of wonder would have likely prompted me to pick the blooms and toss them like minirockets. As an adult, of course, I shudder at the idea. But such an impulse just proves how this extraordinary wildflower ignites the imagination. Such childlike excitement still lives in me when I come upon spring's shooting star, and I marvel in its small wonder.

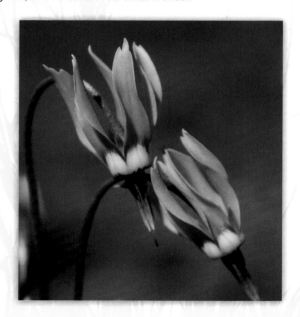

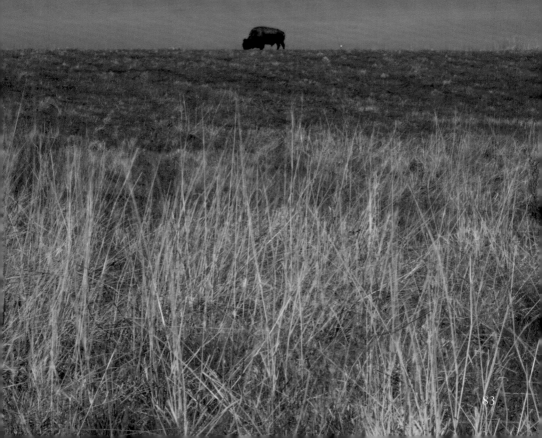

*conversation fifteen*

# MAJESTY

*Thomas Dean*

ere in the Midwest, many often apologize for our landscape. "We don't have any mountains or oceans, but . . ." The American default majestic landscape does not include grasslands. Oh, sure, in the lyrics to "America the Beautiful," "amber waves of grain" do get a callout, but the purple mountains get the "majesties." Even Merriam-Webster, which defines majesty as "greatness or splendor of quality or character," gives as an example "the majesty of the mountains."

But what majesty the prairie holds! We associate "majesty" with splendor, with grandeur, with magnificence. The Middle English sense of "majesty" raises the stakes from Latin's "majus," meaning "major," to invoking, in fact, the greatness of God. Surely that is not the province of only oceans and mountains. Is not an endless green and yellow horizon, with unreachable elevations of swelling cumulus clouds amassed above it, full of anything but grandeur? Are not miles of countless big bluestem turkeyfoot spikes, mingled across the seasons with shades of purple spiderwort, red little bluestem, and ivory rattlesnake master anything but splendorous? Is not a herd of bison—or a lone sentinel—standing proudly on a grassland rise, massive heads in regal contemplation, anything but magnificent?

I know, though, that today's prairie is broken majesty. The broad horizons I enjoy at the Neal Smith National Wildlife Refuge or the Hoover Prairie here in Iowa are measured in acres rather than miles. The restored prairie, raised from disturbed ground, has different proportions of abundance in its grasses and forbs compared to the true native remnant. Very few of the bison remaining in the wild and virtually none in captivity are free of cattle DNA.

Yet I still fully embrace the prairie's broken majesty. I think of "Sparky," the popular bison at Neal Smith Wildlife Refuge, who died this past week as I write. Sparky got his name and popularity from being struck by lightning in 2013, nearly five years before his death. A refuge biologist—the same one who found him dead—discovered the burned and bloodied bison not long after the storm had passed. The folks at Neal Smith were surprised he survived, but visitors to the refuge were always delighted to see the aging bull with the burn scars on his hump lumber past their car on the road. Although Sparky's original majesty was broken, his endurance manifested a different kind of grandeur and inspired awe in all who saw or even just knew of him. Sparky was always majestic, and in many ways grew more so.

If majesty is the greatness of what is beyond our full human comprehension, then it is always unfolding to our senses and understanding. Even when the majesty of the world is broken by human hands—as has been the case for oceans and mountains as well as prairies—nature will find a new path to proclaim its glory. Even when human hands seek to heal the wounds we have laid upon this earth, the splendor that follows is nature's, not our, declamation. Prairie's majesty is always its own.

*Cindy Crosby*

*I* enjoy puzzles. I like the way the full image emerges as I slot each shape into its correct niche. When I slow down and pay attention to the puzzle pieces, I sometimes mentally work through a knotty problem or relationship issue. It's a good process.

But.

One of the most frustrating moments in finishing a thousand-piece puzzle is the realization you lost a piece. Or several pieces. Sure, your image is close. But that one elusive piece keeps the image from what it should be.

That feeling of incompleteness nags you.

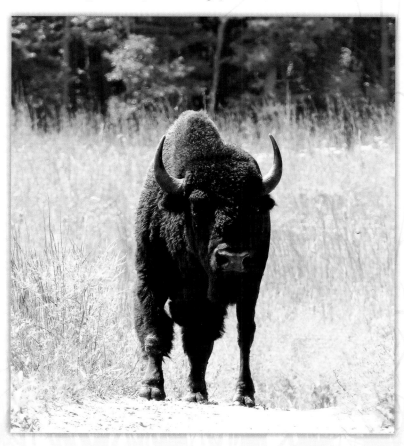

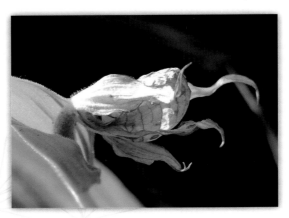

I think of this as I hike Nachusa Grasslands, a four-thousand-acre site managed by the Nature Conservancy in Illinois. Nachusa Grasslands is tucked into a patchwork quilt of farms about ninety miles west of downtown Chicago. Over its twenty-plus-year history of restoring habitat, Nachusa Grasslands has served as host to more than seven hundred native plant species, about two hundred kinds of birds, and countless amphibians, insects, reptiles, and mammals. Orchids and ornate box turtles. Dazzling dragonflies and dickcissels. Slithery snakes and shooting star wildflowers.

It seems like enough species to make a majestic image, doesn't it? And yet.

A piece of the puzzle was missing here. A big piece.

*Bison bison.* That's the scientific name. We know them more commonly as "American buffalo." They disappeared from Illinois early in the 1800s. But since 2014, through the efforts of people who aren't afraid to dream big, they are at Nachusa Grasslands.

When I first began as a steward at Nachusa and heard about the plan to restore bison, I wondered. Would the preserve suddenly seem like a zoo? Or one of those exotic animal farms you drive by in rural areas—you know the ones—full of zebras and llamas and ostrich? A curiosity?

When the first bison were trucked in and lumbered out into the tallgrass to graze, my fears were assuaged. Just as a puzzle has a gaping hole where a missing piece should have fit, I realized Nachusa had always been incomplete . . . until now.

Conservationist Aldo Leopold wrote, "To keep every cog and wheel is the first precaution of intelligent tinkering." We almost lost the bison in North America. And if we had, the tallgrass prairie restoration puzzle would always seem incomplete.

The grazing bison silhouetted against the setting sun look majestic today at Nachusa Grasslands, and other preserves where they have been restored, such as Midewin National Tallgrass Prairie just south of Chicago. A seamless part of the prairie landscape.

Like they belong there.

As they do.

# DIVERSITY

*Cindy Crosby*

"What are we made of? How did the universe begin?"

At Fermilab, the nation's "premier particle physics laboratory," advanced particle accelerators help its seventeen hundred scientists and researchers "dig down to the smallest building blocks of matter" and "probe the farthest reaches of the universe." As an outpost of the United States Department of Energy here in Illinois, it is heavily protected by guards during times of national crisis such as 9/11. Today I am free to hike Fermilab's hundreds of acres of restored prairie and trails. I show the gate guard my driver's license, and he waves me through.

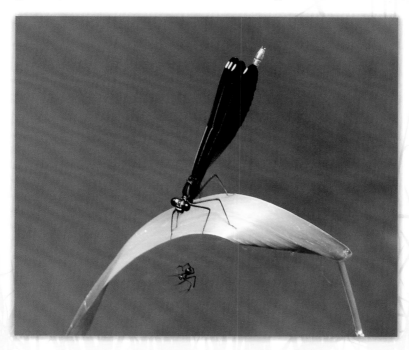

The past and the future collide here, much as the particles in the accelerator ring once collided not far from my path. "Our vision is to solve the mysteries of matter, energy, space and time for the benefit of all," reads their creed of faith. I admire the work these scientists do; I understand their drive to *know*. The greater drive I feel, however, is to make my peace with unsolved mysteries, even while reaching for understanding.

The trails across the prairie stretch to the horizon line, unbroken except by the occasional scrubby tree. And a large pile of . . . something.

I hike that way. It appears a tornado has swept through a woodland, then tossed everything into the tallgrass. Tree after tree after tree stacked on the prairie like pixie sticks, taller than my head. Cut and piled—to be burned? Chipped for wood paths? I wonder. Why would anyone advocate this wholesale destruction?

I look closer. Ah! This particular mystery is solved.

Ash trees.

The ash trees in the Chicago region have been decimated by a tiny pest: the emerald ash borer. The trees are weakened and then die as the ash borer moves from tree to tree; street to street; from woodland to woodland, from state to state. Only stumps remain of what once were beautiful, stately trees, valued for their utility, their shade, and their beauty.

A way of life as we know it is passing. Imagine a world without trees? I never could, until this.

In 2015, my suburban Chicago subdivision's streets were lined with beautiful, mature ash trees. By 2017, they were all dead. Our neighborhood

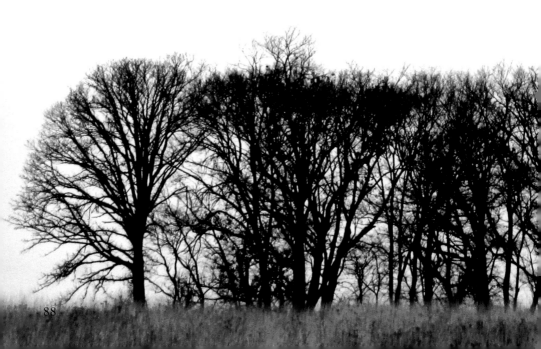

parkway was a virtual desert. Historically, we planted rows of American elm trees in the same way as we planted ash in the 1960s. Both ash and elm were an easy choice for the developers of communities—economical, beautiful. Why choose anything else?

When we commit to the easy way—planting one kind of anything—we gamble. It is simpler, isn't it, to know and promote only a few flowers or trees or grasses for our landscape? We know what they will look like, their requirements and habits. It's more comfortable. A no-brainer. But when we do, we lose the benefits of a vibrant, healthy landscape teeming with different trees, plants, and their associated animals, birds, and insects. We lose diversity.

As the emerald ash borers moved from tree to tree, they left hieroglyphics. Peel the bark back, and you'll see the marks. These are known as the "gallery." And indeed, it is artwork of a certain type. I imagine the message of the ash borer hieroglyphics is this: *Embrace diversity.* Think about how to make life richer, not easier.

I hike the prairie past the corpses of the ash trees. My grandchildren will never know what they lost. But I know that there is a hole in the natural world that nothing else will fill, just as my great-grandparents knew what a world with the American chestnut looked like and mourned its loss.

By refusing to acknowledge our need for diversity, what else will we lose?

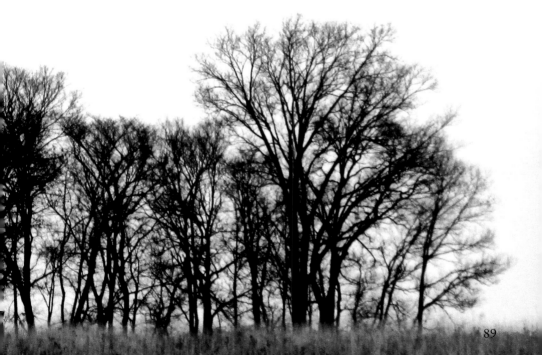

89

*Thomas Dean*

iversity on the prairie also depends on what's above.

The prairie ecosystem is among the most diverse on the planet. As Paul Gruchow tells us in "What the Prairie Teaches Us" in his paragraph on the grassland's diversity, "One hundred acres of prairie may support three thousand species of insects alone, each of them poised to exploit—often beneficially—certain plants, microclimates, soils, weather conditions, and seasons." The key to ecological health is interdependence, and diversity is key to interdependence.

The prairie's diversity also makes a visit a true personal pleasure, providing so much to see and experience whether you're there as a naturalist, a hiker, an artist, or someone who just needs a dose of nature. Those with some knowledge of how the prairie works understand that what we see isn't all of what we get. The majority of the prairie's mass—even the most important aspects of its lifeblood—lies in the deep, deep roots underground.

But we shouldn't look only in front of our noses and down at (and beyond) our feet to know and appreciate prairie diversity. We should also look up—to the broad sky above. Few other landscapes on earth offer such an unobstructed view of the sky, which itself is elemental to the prairie experience. And that sky only deepens the diversity of the prairie experience.

A totally clear day allows the yellows of compass plants and sunflowers to glow against the deep blue sky in glorious ways.

Wisps of cirrus clouds subtly complement the delicacy of waving bluestem.

Cumulus piling higher and higher reminds us of the dynamic magnitude of this land.

Sunrise and sunset can set the sky ablaze in astonishing pinks, oranges, and purples that shine a whole new light (so to speak) on what sometimes has become a familiar sight.

Overcast gray flattens the individual plants competing for our attention, revealing the prairie as a singular entity as well as a collective of many distinct beings.

When the mists and rains descend, land and sky merge, melding into a special oneness that ladles life-giving liquid onto the tallgrass.

And when the cumulonimbus lowers into a wall cloud, thunder cracks and lightning strikes, and the sky may bring regenerating fire to the grasses and forbs.

Sun, wind, and water combine to make the sky a dynamic entity unto itself as well as a kaleidoscopic keystone in the ecology of the prairie. The grassland's diversity of life could not exist without the diversity of the sky, and the palette of our prairie experience is much the richer for it.

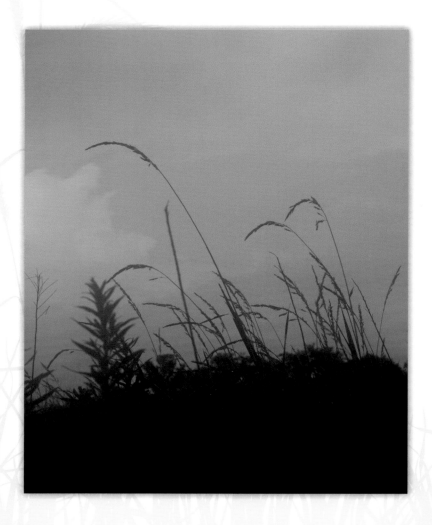

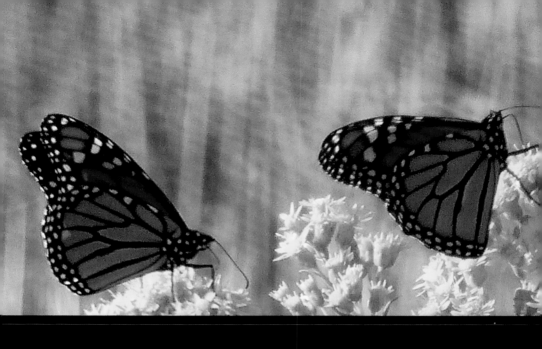

the *spirit of*

REFLECTION

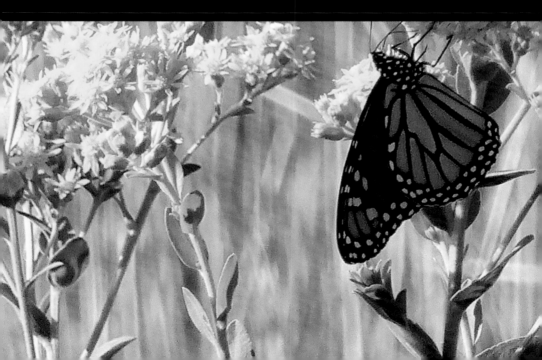

# DESIGN

*Thomas Dean*

On the winter prairie
Design remains

Color fades
Seed drops
Petal withers
Leaf unmoors

But bluestem's stalk still bends
Blazing star's scaffold still stands
Silphium's architecture still holds
Oak's arms still reach skyward
All in winter's still song

On the winter prairie
Shadows play
Fears fall
The path clarifies
Purpose stands
Design remains

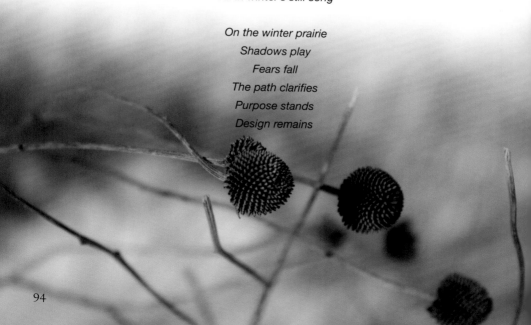

*Cindy Crosby*

T he artist Georgia O'Keeffe noted, "When you take a flower in your hand and really look at it, it's your world for the moment."

It's early spring, and I'm sitting on a small hill under the trees, looking out over the prairie. Not much is up on the prairie proper—a little pale Indian plantain, the first flush of wood betony and violets. But here in the savanna is a colony of bloodroot. I count the flowers—a single bloom per plant—and stop around five hundred.

I put away my phone and my camera, feeling like I'm about to fly somewhere ("Please turn off all electronic devices. . . ."). Indeed, all around me, flight is in progress. The pollinators are making Chicago's O'Hare International Airport look quiet. There's the flash and whir of wings, the buzz and purr of insect life scouting for sustenance. Exactly the way it should be.

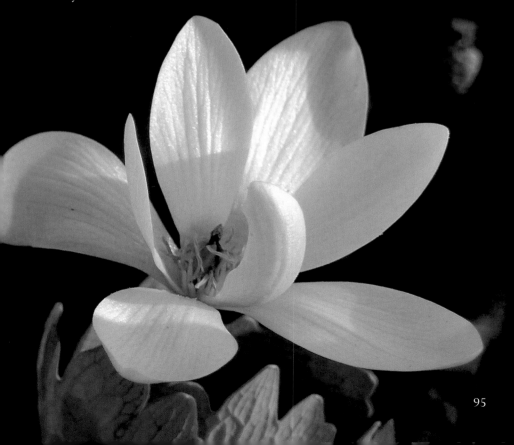

If you want to really see the prairie, break out your sketch pad. Find a comfortable place to sit. Look at the amazing natural designs all around you. Then focus on a single plant for an hour. I choose one bloodroot bud to sketch and, to my amazement, watch it unfold over the course of about a minute. Who knew? Not me. Not until I gave it my single-minded attention.

What other wonders am I missing?

In this early season, bloodroot has adapted to hedge its bets. It's designed to ensure survival. A thoughtful article by W. John Hayden from Richmond University explains the bloodroot model: "Hurry, wait, and hedge against uncertain fate." Then, he goes on to describe the process. The bloodroot pushes out blooms before much else is in evidence on the prairie edge. The first day, it opens wide, waiting for early bees to check it out. Potential pollinators will be disappointed—there is no nectar reward—but will carry off a load of pollen. On the second day, the bloodroot opens again. Waiting for pollinators.

But given the dicey weather in the Chicago region—and bloodroot's propensity to close in cloudy, drizzly, cold conditions and at night—the pollinator "window" might be mostly closed. So on day three, the blood-root employs a desperation strategy. The anthers bend inward toward the style instead of outward, and the flower self-pollinates. That and some strategic rhizonomous reproduction ensure large colonies of bloodroot for years to come.

The astonishing complexity and smart strategies of a single wildflower make me realize the overwhelming majesty of the prairie—and our world. What design! It's enough to bring you to your knees.

Why not put this book down, take a moment, and go see?

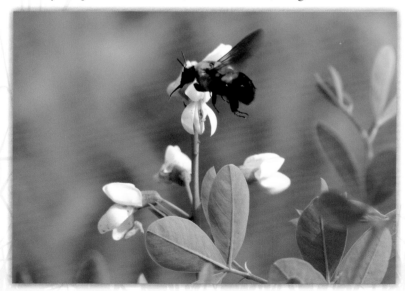

# LINES

*Thomas Dean*

*Axis mundi!*
*Center of the world! Navel of the earth!*
*The line from sky to earth to soil,*
*conduit between cosmic spirit and manifest nature.*

*Horizon!*
*Broad expanse of earth's skin! Plane of the planet's stage!*
*The line from east to west, from north to south,*
*impelling creation's power to the four directions.*

*Prairie!*
*Dais for earth's broadest lines!*
*Juncture of universal and terrestrial powers!*
*The line its essence, yet the curve of the world bending*
*its force and splendor back into me.*

*Cindy Crosby*

Sometimes the familiar looks unfamiliar. Winter—and fire—have this effect on the prairie.

When cold weather sets in, the prairie undergoes a transformation. Greens of every possible hue are replaced by metallics—golds, grays, rusts. Stripped of lush leaves and drained of color, wildflowers take on a new look. Their scaffolding—stems holding up seedheads—are in the spotlight.

Squiggles and tunnels in the snow are evidence of vole movements. A series of parallel lines brushed into one snowdrift, plus some feathers, tells the story of a battle between a red-tailed hawk and a small bird. The lines of this story are as old as time—the hunter and the hunted, the predator and the prey.

When we set a prescribed fire, the prairie changes in a matter of hours. Trail lines suddenly appear, previously invisible for months under dense vegetation. Anthills pop up from nowhere. Critter tunnels lie exposed in the newly burned earth.

You can see the deep gouges and gullies where water runs fast and deep across the prairie in a downpour. Old survey markers show up, as do agricultural relics, left over from the days when this prairie was farmed.

As I grow older, my face is becoming creased and wrinkled. There are lines everywhere—crow's feet at the corners of my eyes where I've squinted into the sun for season after season, lines around my mouth from smiling and frowning. My emotions are writ large upon my face with these lines.

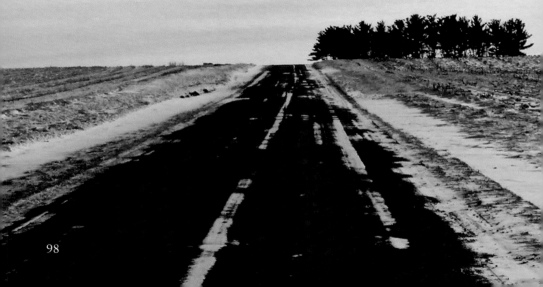

The prairie and I both share this: our lines show the progression of years, the events of the past, the stories that are still being written today. Each line is evidence of life being fully lived. Without the distractions of youth—a smooth face; a more sculpted, agile body—my "scaffolding"—the underlying true self I've been striving toward for more than fifty years—is much more in the forefront these days.

Prairie lines are about weather, creatures, fire. They tell the story of a place. My lines tell of laughter, of suffering, of good times and bad times, of time spent outdoors. They tell the story of my life.

Our society abhors any sign of age. Yet I try to embrace what's written on my face, just as I read the lines written on the prairie. Both of our lines show evidence that life is being fully lived. Both show that we are survivors in a world that can be a tough place.

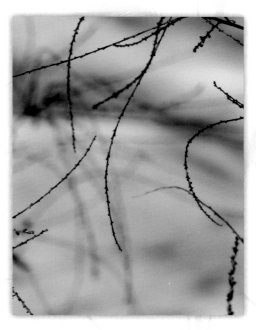

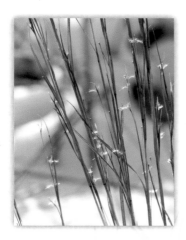

# DIRECTION

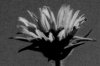

*Thomas Dean*

*I* wander the late July prairie. The compass plant calls my eyes upward to its full eight feet above the summer grasses and wildflowers. It stands silent, strong, undisturbed as the breeze rustles the bluestem. The sunburst yellow flowers sit in their delicacy atop the sturdy stalk. Hugging the stem close, fuzzy-rough and deepening green leaves have turned their spiky points upward. I can't see their movement in time, but they are turning like clock hands, seeking the sky and then north and south to protect themselves from the burning midday sun. As they did for the pioneers, these leaves provide me direction, inviting me to find my place in the prairie.

For the European prairie pioneers, the compass plant was a stay against disorientation. Lost in an endless sea of grasses with no landmarks to guide them, those seeking a new land or a new home, or simply passage through, looked to the tall stems with the small sunflowers rising above all else. The pioneers would direct their attention to the large, spiky leaves on the hairy stem to recenter, to reorient, to find north and south once again.

Today, *we* live disoriented, perhaps more completely than the pioneers who lost momentary sense of which way to go. Today, we have lost our way by disconnecting from the cycles of life and the workings of the earth. We claim license to dominate rather than adapt to nature, to alter our habitat for an artificial vision that ignores the life of the true world.

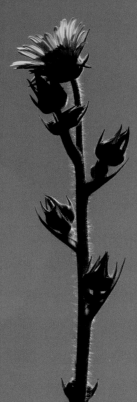
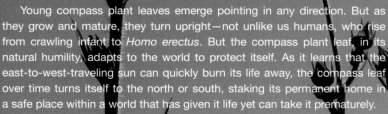

Young compass plant leaves emerge pointing in any direction. But as they grow and mature, they turn upright—not unlike us humans, who rise from crawling infant to *Homo erectus*. But the compass plant leaf, in its natural humility, adapts to the world to protect itself. As it learns that the east-to-west-traveling sun can quickly burn its life away, the compass leaf over time turns itself to the north or south, staking its permanent home in a safe place within a world that has given it life yet can take it prematurely.

I imagine a world where humans have learned the lesson of the compass plant—not just how to find north and south, but the deeper lesson, the lesson of directing ourselves to live abundantly and safely in this world of awesome beauty and great powers, the lesson of humility: to adapt and honor rather than dominate and destroy. Our true north points not toward a land we can exploit but dwells in a natural home where we thrive, and where we understand and care for the world that gives us life. I also imagine that in our thriving, understanding, and caring, the compass plant will respond by once again rising from the grasses, standing regal sentinel across millions of acres of natural prairie, guiding us still in the direction of living well and rightly on this earth.

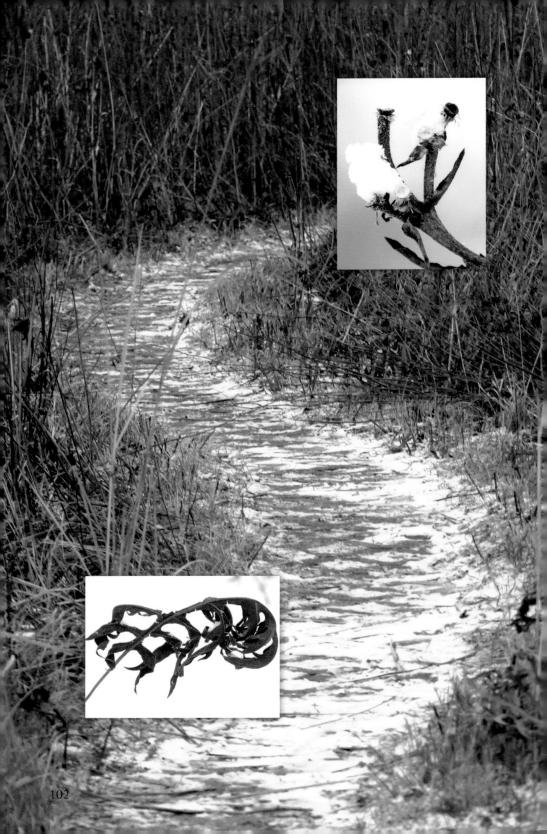

*Cindy Crosby*

Compass Plant

*Come.*
*I know which way to go*
*I've spent my life pointing*
*Everyone in the right direction.*

*It is good to be so certain*
*So decidedly right*
*It rids you of unnecessary*
*Anxiety, worries, indecision*
*Like, what about this way?*
*Take this road? That one?*
*Maybe just sit down . . .*
*or Risk?*
*Risk?*
*Risk?*

*Deeply rooted in my confidence*
*I tell you*
*Go here.*
*It is the proper path.*
*Do not turn from it.*

*If you choose badly*
*It is only because*
*You did not listen.*

*If I tell you the right direction to go, then,*
*Why, oh why*
*Do you keep asking*
*These endless questions?*

*conversation twenty*

# MYSTERY

*Thomas Dean*

Sometimes when I'm on the prairie, its mystery overwhelms me, yet that is when I try most earnestly to call to it. The invocation to mystery can come when fog drapes the grasses, or when sunset draws long shadows across the broad prairie and paints the wildflowers in black silhouette. Sometimes mystery comes when my attention is pulled into an infinite microworld inside a raindrop nestled in the fold of a long bluestem leaf. Sometimes it even comes in the midst of bright, bold clarity that pours across the colorful expanse of yellow *Silphium* under sunny high pressure. No matter when or where it happens, the mystery of prairie always presents to me as questions.

Is the mystery in a mythic wholeness, an eternal return where all time exists simultaneously amongst the deep roots and rhizomes, where original native and ecological restoration become one?

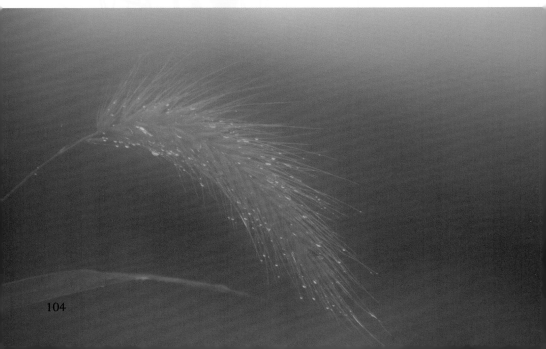

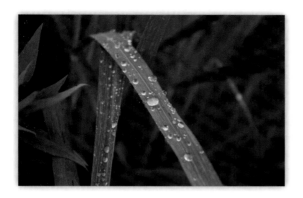

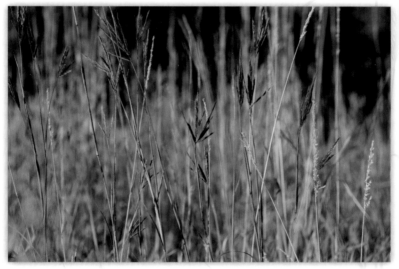

Is the mystery coming from the voices of peoples and histories buried under the earth that continues to spring forth with new life?

Is it in the intricacies and richness of a magnificent ecosystem that I just cannot fully comprehend? Or is it simply in my own ignorance of how all iterations of fluttering side oats grama, fanciful Turk's cap, and boastful red-winged blackbird embrace each other in interdependence?

Is the prairie a mask or a revelation? Does it wish to shield me from its incomprehensible truth or disclose to me the powers of compass plant and bergamot that push my understanding?

I realize these questions are not enquiries to be answered but invitations to lose myself in the greater whole that is prairie, and the world. They pave the way for the humility required of me to offer ethical care and appropriate honor. How little I know. How little I understand. I accept the mystery, and I accept the prairie. I hope it accepts me.

*Cindy Crosby*

I'm a big fan of mysteries. As a teenager, I burned through all of Agatha Christie's classics, and I still love to pick up an occasional thriller that keeps me guessing. As a naturalist, part of my attraction to the outdoors revolves around a different sort of mystery. Science has a lot of answers. But there are many unsolved questions out there. The prairie is full of them. Perhaps nowhere is mystery so evident as when I try to understand dragonfly migration.

Every spring, I train dragonfly monitors to collect data at the prairies where I'm a steward. We're all volunteers, all citizen scientists collecting information that we hope will help future researchers learn more about these incredible insects. During the workshops, we'll discuss the life cycle of the dragonfly. We'll share ID tips for differentiating among the 150 or so dragonfly and damselfly species found in our little corner of the Midwest, plus the variations among male, female, and immature individuals. Pretty straightforward stuff, for the most part. Dragonfly cultural history and much of dragonfly natural history is explainable, at least to some degree.

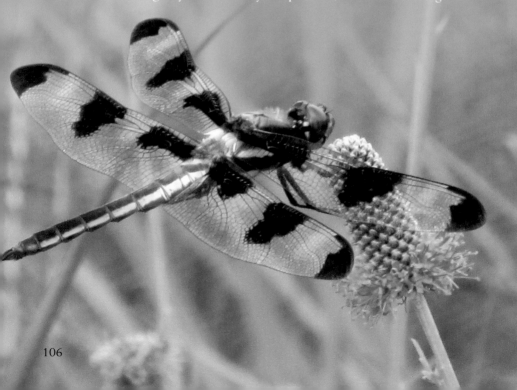

But dragonfly migration! That's where explanations get difficult. "Instinct is a marvelous thing. It can neither be explained nor ignored," wrote Agatha Christie.

Dragonfly migration is less understood than that of the monarch butterfly, whose travel habits have been exhaustively studied and immortalized in books, and whose migration journey continues to fascinate the general public. Or consider bird migration, the topic of many books and the subject of countless research projects. Sure, there's still mystery in avian migration. But plenty of information is out there.

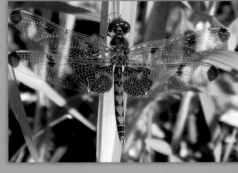

Dragonfly migration? Not so much. The process remains veiled in mystery. We do know a few things: at least four dragonfly species in the Midwest (green darner, black saddlebags, wandering glider, and variegated meadowhawk) head south for the winter, and probably others as well. But why these species? Why not others? Where do they go? What tells them to mass at the end of summer and fly, often in large swarms, to another place?

We know that some dragonflies in North America may travel almost two thousand miles south in the late summer and early fall. Dragonfly offspring will travel the same distances, often with raptors, back north in the spring. Look around in science journals and on dragonfly websites and you'll find comical images of green darners wearing tiny transmitters to track their movements. Complex studies of isotopes in dragonfly wings help researchers determine their general place of emergence.

In April, we'll begin to see the first battered and worn-out dragonflies arrive in the Midwest, heirs of those stalwart flyers who fled south last year. As dragonfly monitors, we'll scribble about these early arrivals—and later, summer flyers and dragonfly departures—as hash marks on our data sheets. We'll report the information to our local and state dragonfly organizations. All very logical and linear, isn't it?

But at some point in the season, most of us will put our clipboards and pencils down and pause for a moment. Overcome with wonder. How amazing that this tiny creature logged those miles and survived birds, weather, and traffic to be here, on this prairie! How incredible that we can bear witness to this phenomenon even for a moment. How satisfying to be a small cog in the wheel of the research that is being done for the future!

Most of us will acknowledge this: despite the data we'll collect, despite all the facts we know, it's the unknown that makes it so exciting to be a part of this citizen science project. The quest is part of the fun.

We'll marvel, in awe of the mystery of dragonfly migration.

107

# DEPTH

*Thomas Dean*

*W*inter is the foundation of the prairie's story, its annual journey around the sun. While not the showiest, the time of dark and cold tells perhaps the most essential chapter of all the seasons.

A good story brings us into an experience. Before we are brought out of it wiser and changed, we encounter intensity, conflict, sometimes danger, and, if the story is worthy, beauty. Of all the seasons, we journey into and out of winter most consciously and intentionally. I am most fulfilled when I feel all the dimensions of this story deeply. The more cold and snow, the more we know we are in deep, unmistakably in a place and time that does not resemble where we entered or where we will exit.

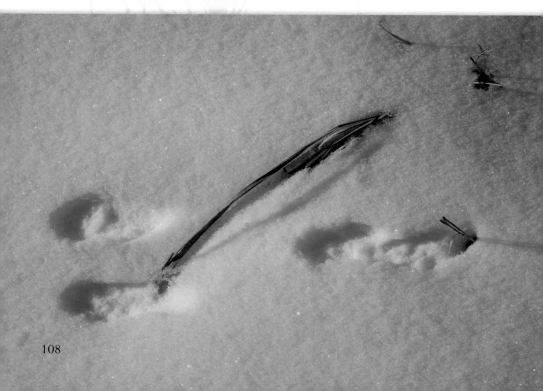

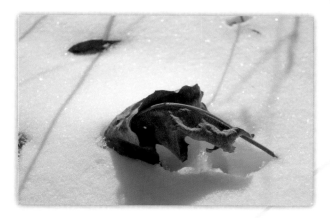

In the prairie's story, winter is a quiet time, when dormancy reigns. Prairie dock leaves brown, shrink, and sag. The bluestem remains tall, but it yellows and turns brittle as its quickening fades. Wild indigo's pods dry and hollow out. As the wind sweeps over the grassland, the sounds of swaying grasses and disturbed husks and hulls are subtle and crisp. No birds sing to the percussive ostinato.

Yet on the winter prairie, life gathers its force to emerge and then explode in vernal epitasis. As the deep snow smothers the past year's growth, its moist blanket broods over the next year's life patiently rejuvenating below in the rich, deep, and dark soil.

In winter, we are much like the prairie's subterra and supraterra. We slacken and perhaps droop, but in our rest, we are recharging our *élan vital*. The more in deep we are, the more our own life stories lengthen their roots, the more vibrant is our emergence in spring.

Nature's fury may overwhelm us with a monumental blizzard, ice storm, or subzero Arctic blast. These are the narrative twists and turns that a good story spawns. When we reach the end of such a tale, even a harrowing one, our protagonist is wiser and perhaps triumphant, as are we. A good winter should make us feel the same way come April.

But winter gifts us not only with harshness and trials. On the prairie, if we cannot perceive the gorgeousness of a resilient compass plant stalk standing lonely sentry in the quietness of a heavy snowfall, or the stark exquisiteness of bare oak branches rising from a savanna against a steel-gray sky, or the awesome misty breath of a harsh wind blowing over a fallow sea of Indian grass, then our aesthetic palette needs revitalizing from a good winter's tale.

Winter on the prairie is a beautiful and frightening story. We will emerge at the denouement, perhaps blinking our eyes after the darkness or raising our arms toward the sun's warmth as we wander the green-up and delight at the first pasque flower. But to get there, we—and the prairie—must first be in deep, letting the tale grow on its own terms, in its own time, and within its own beauty.

*Cindy Crosby*

Visit the two prairies where I'm a steward in the summer months, and it's a visual feast for the eyes. Regal fritillary butterflies and amber-wing dragonflies jostle for position on butter-yellow prairie coreopsis, pale purple coneflowers, and silver-globed rattlesnake master. The bright greens of the grasses stretch from horizon to horizon.

But winter. That's a different story.

Take a hike on the prairie in January or February when the tallgrass is flattened and drained of color. Dead leaves and seedheads litter the landscape. To most people, it may not look like much. Shallow. Ugly.

I've learned the hard way that the end of winter is not great for that first introduction to prairie for friends and visitors. What I see through a lens of love, others might see as an old snow-covered field. Or simply a mess.

Understanding this was a turning point for me in how I explained my passion for prairies and other natural areas and their communities to friends. I realized that without spending time in a place, many family members and acquaintances couldn't be expected to understand why I invested thousands of hours hiking, sweating, teaching, planning, and collecting data about a place that, on the surface, looked a bit wild and messy to the untrained eye.

Without knowing that the deep prairie roots wait under the soil, ready to explode with grasses and wildflowers in the spring, you might not find a lot to get excited about.

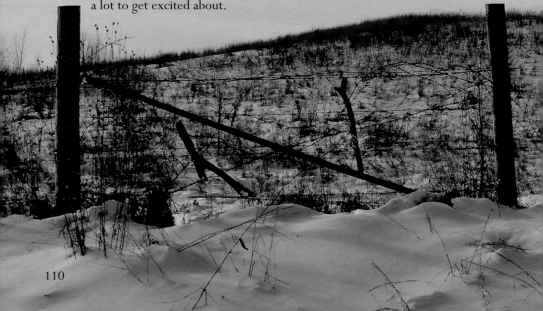

My steward fieldwork—pulling weeds, collecting native prairie seeds, monitoring for dragonflies and damselflies—has brought me into a close relationship with the tallgrass prairie. But without this kind of relationship to the land, I have to remember other people will not necessarily see the prairie with the same wonder, joy, and anticipation that I do.

People ask me, "Why does it take so much work? Can't you just let nature do its thing and leave the tallgrass alone?" Visitors come to the prairie with buckets to pick the "weeds" for their dinner party table arrangements. Others cringe when a dragonfly buzzes by. "Won't it sting me?"

As someone who came to fieldwork later in life, I remember how it felt to see only "weeds" or "bugs" or even just a snowy old field with some dead leaves. I had the same questions. I'm reminded of the different ways I need to find to connect hearts and minds with the prairie I love.

It's all about showing up each week to do whatever task needs to be done. Seeing the prairie and its creatures in all sorts of weather, in different seasons, and at various times of day. Reading a book about prairie. Taking a class. Exploring the tallgrass with all five senses. Building a relationship with a place.

Deep relationships are about spending time with someone or something, then sharing what you love with others. Supporting the science. Changing public policy because you care. Building relationships. Taking care of our landscape of home. Going deep.

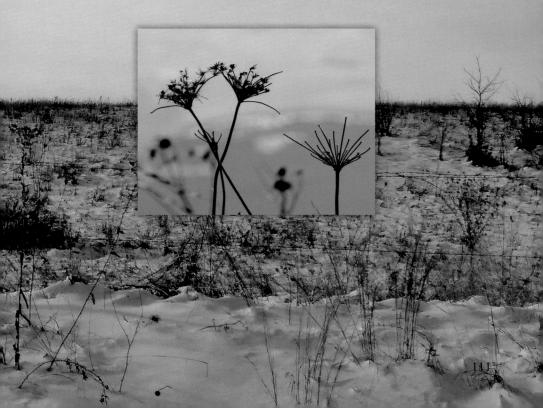

# SHADOW

*Thomas Dean*

In Plato's allegory of the cave, chained prisoners see only shadows cast onto the rock wall before them, shadows created by people and objects passing by a fire behind them. Many interpret the prisoners to be the human race, unable to see Plato's Forms (or Ideas) beyond the limitations of our human senses.

On the prairie, shadows expand rather than limit vision. As poet David Whyte tells us, a shadow reflects presence, not absence. As the sun's rays lengthen in summer's late afternoon, the prairie dock leaf turns translucent, like a Javanese *wayang kulit* puppet theater screen, revealing the delicate, spare shapes of wildflowers standing behind it. As the autumn sun dips below the horizon at dusk, its fingers of light project upward, turning the grasses and forbs dark to my eyes, making of them silhouettes, shadow's sibling. In winter's cold, the sunlight above projects the outline of a bent goldenrod stem onto the ground's snowy surface, reminding me that I can see nothing more below, not even the surface soil on which leaves lie dormant and under which roots grow deep and microbes flourish.

These dark shapes, delicate black lines and efflorescences, carry with them their own beauty—the presence not just of the barely seen, but that of their own essential design on a two-dimensional field.

Despite their intrinsic beauty, the prairie shadows remind me that my sight is limited, but unlike the prisoners in the cave, they arouse in me not hopelessness and helplessness in my ignorance, but joy and humility in my privilege to be present here. Contrary to their two-dimensional monochromaticism, shadows afford awareness of depth, of substance, of dimension.

The prairie is a world of immense variety, shape, texture—substances *and* forms—that are in the end not entirely knowable. Like the flickering outlines on the cave wall, the prairie shadows tell us there is so much more we cannot see. But that message does not imprison us. Rather, it invites us to explore, to learn, and to experience to the greatest extent we can, yet also to marvel at what we will never fully apprehend.

I would grieve living in a world without shadows, in large part because I would understand the prairie so much less without them.

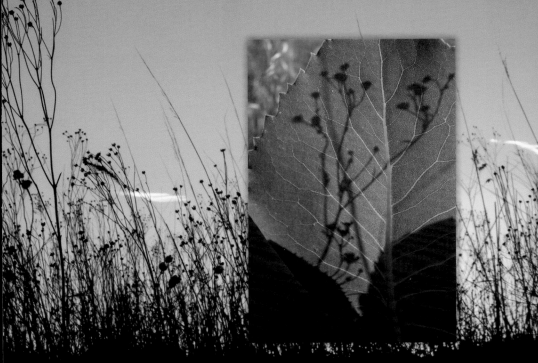

*Cindy Crosby*

It's "shadow season" on the prairie—too warm for winter, too cold for spring, when everything seems a ghost of its former vibrant self. I find it one of the most difficult times of the year in the tallgrass. Everything that remains at the turn of March to April is seemingly brittle. Ruined. Grasses are flattened. The prairie seems worn out.

Waiting for fire.

Or maybe I'm just projecting my own winter-weary self on the prairie. The prairie—as always—has its gifts to give. These gifts just aren't that in-your-face, "wow-look-at-that-color!" good looks. No wildflowers. No juicy grasses. Few returning grassland birds. There is a whole lot of animal scat and mud. Trash. Flotsam and jetsam left behind after the snow melt.

It's discouraging. But sometimes, to see hope for the future—or even just to give yourself a mental boost to get to next week—you have to look a little closer. Dig a little deeper. Take more time. Sit with things. When you do, you find that with the prairie's maturity comes a different sort of beauty.

It's nuanced. Prairie dock leaves are so wrinkled, you have to look twice to recognize them. Much different from their beginnings less than a year or so ago. All the knowledge of the past prairie season is encapsulated here in March. A shadow of what once was. You can't help but be reminded of our own fleeting presence on Earth.

There's promise. That promise will be more evident after the prescribed fires, when the prairie is once again lush and green and beginning to bloom.

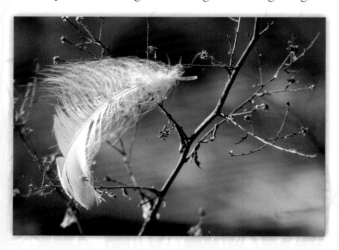

Despite the stands of dead foliage, what is important to the prairie is still here. Even if unseen. It's right where you're standing. Down deep where the fire can't touch it, in the roots that plunge up to fifteen feet or more into the earth.

Martin Luther King Jr. said, "Everything we see is but a shadow cast by that which we don't see." He wasn't talking about the prairie, but his words are applicable. Those unseen deep roots that grip the soil so tenaciously—and that will remain untouched by fire—are the prairie's future. They hold the history of the prairie and its soil in their grasp. While the life of the prairie above the ground is finished—that fleeting shadow of wildflowers, grasses, and color—there is more to consider than what is visible to our eyes.

Some prairies have already been burned as March comes to a close. But without the right weather conditions, many of our local prairies remain in a state of anticipation. Waiting for the flames. For the prairie to flourish—for color and life and motion to be kindled again in the tallgrass—calls for something harsh, extravagant, and radical to happen.

Bring on the fire.

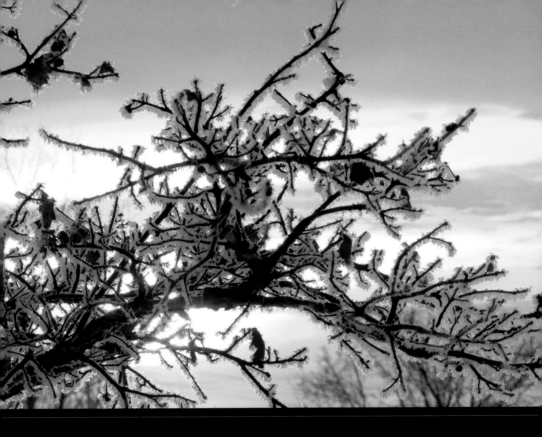

the spirit of

HOPE

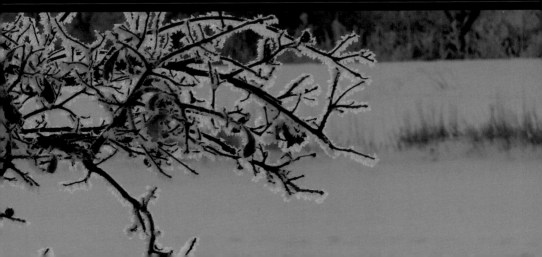

*conversation twenty-three*

# TRANSITIONS

*Cindy Crosby*

*J*anuary's vivid prairie sunsets remind me of the black light posters I had in the early seventies. Pow! Unbelievable colors. You wouldn't expect this kind of show in a landscape you thought had gone all taupe grasses and gray skies.

What amazements winter pulls out of her bag of tricks! The whims and vagaries of weather in January bring about both ice and thaw. My backyard prairie pond glasses in plants and leaves.

Down in the still-frozen shallows of Willoway Brook on the Schulenberg Prairie, the broken stalks of white wild indigo lie tangled up in blue snow shadows. Along the streambank, milkweed pods stand ready to serve as makeshift boats. Spilled of their floss, they could float downstream in a thaw, sailing a million miles away.

My mind seems to drift off that far in January sometimes as well. Anything seems possible.

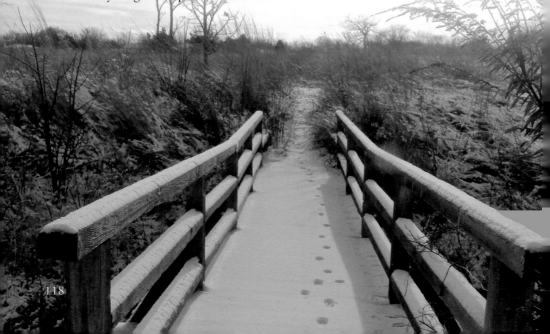

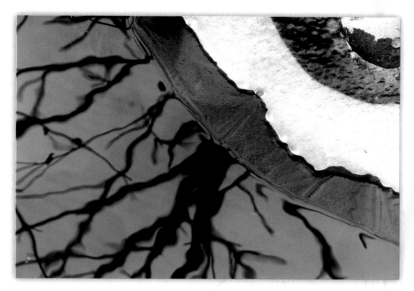

Where the current runs deep in the stream, there's open water. So much tension! The muscle of ice against flow; the push and pull of solid to liquid. Transitions.

I always find transitions difficult. But they often signal some sort of breakthrough. January is a good moment to pause and reflect on this. Be encouraged instead of discouraged by these passages, these changes.

Meanwhile, Willoway Brook wrestles with its own transitions. Ice splinters and fractures. Shards tumble downstream. The water sings of spring on the way.

*Soon. Soon.*

The ice, cold and slick, is a foil for the other sensory pleasures of the prairie this month. Today it's bright sun. Tomorrow it might be a shroud of fog across the grasses.

Breathe in, and you inhale the scent of evaporating snow in the air. Lean down and touch a rasp of sandpapery compass plant leaf. Listen to the castanet rattle of milkvetch pods, holed by insects, each with its cache of dry seeds beating time in the breeze. Listen! In the clear air of January, sound seems to travel a little farther than in other months.

The brittle and the rough stand in sharp contrast to the last soft brushes of little bluestem, still holding rich color in the otherwise bleached-out grasses.

All of these pleasures add joy to January's hours. The ever-present geese honk their lane changes overhead against a backdrop of jet contrails that crisscross the sky. Each day—as the sun burns its way up through the east and then falls in flames to the west—you know the cycle of freeze–thaw, freeze–thaw brings spring a little closer. That's a transition to anticipate.

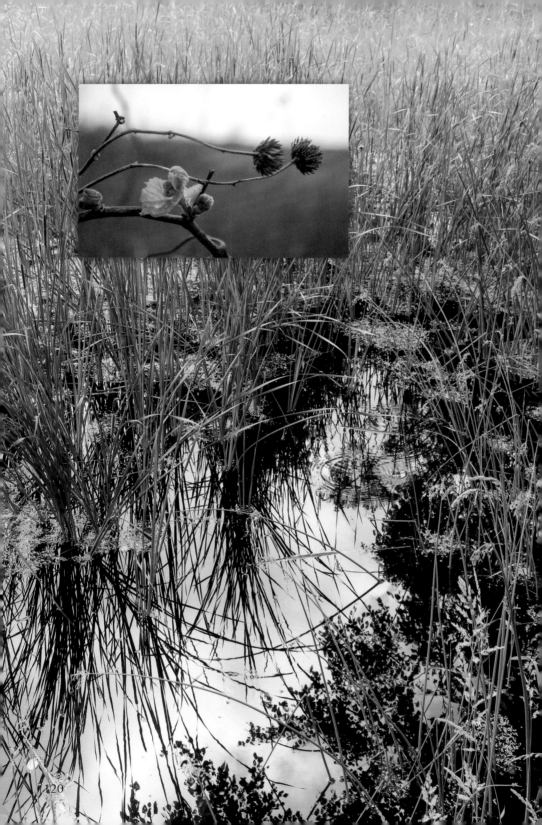

*Thomas Dean*

*April is small,*
*But it is rising.*

*The taut, reedy chorus frog song is rising*
*Up its scale to the stars.*
*The creek water, still shallow, is rising*
*After last night's rain.*
*The bluestem is rising green and spare,*
*Infant spears among the yellowed elder stalks.*

*The prairie grass is rising from mud,*
*Held deep for its upward journey to light*
*By waking roots, long, wide, and wise from time.*
*In April, we are small,*
*But we are rising,*
*Emerging from the humus, where lies*
*The dilating humility of our unseen beginning.*

*We ask of ourselves the same we ask of*
*The grass, the flower, the tree, the frog, the water—*
*How high?*
*How wide?*
*How deep?*
*How colorful?*
*How beautiful.*

# CHANGE

*Cindy Crosby*

*I* open the window and lean against it, inhaling the cool, moist air and listening to the rain outside. Spring is here, and with it the sounds of renewal.

But there is something else besides the tapping of raindrops. *Creak! Creak!* Like a rusty door hinge. It is a western chorus frog, who has found his way to my tiny hand-dug backyard prairie pond and is calling for a mate. It's a lonely sound, with no response in the rain. But he doesn't give up.

After a while, as much as I enjoy frogs, I find myself longing for an off switch. Even with the window shut, his voice is there—*creakkkkkk*—over and over in the background.

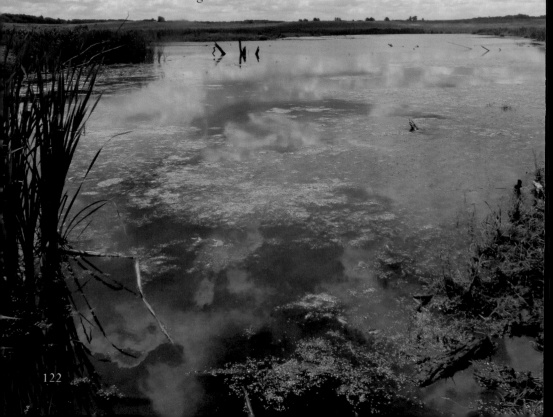

My handkerchief of a yard is surrounded on all four sides by modern homes. Privacy is a desired commodity. I have listened to these frogs and their counterparts, the spring peepers, as I hike the prairie wetlands. I love the summer songs of American bullfrogs and green frogs as well. But I have never had western chorus frogs in my pond before.

When we moved here, I willingly dug through the hard clay to create this little pool of water. I knew that water is an invitation. It speaks of something bigger than myself. It invites a loss of control. It shows a willingness to embrace mystery. The prairie pond fills and dries, overflows and goes empty with the fickle nature of Illinois weather. In winter it is a small ice rink dusted with snow that shows me the passage of winter animals and birds.

On fine spring mornings, I find muddy footprints all around the pond and across the concrete patio: a raccoon pausing to wash its supper; a fox, sometimes glimpsed as we are working in the yard, stopping for a drink; two mallard ducks flying in for a short swim.

The tiny pond reminds me that if I prepare a place where I give up control of what I want to see and instead see what comes, it will not always be pretty like the dragonflies. Water is an invitation for change. Some of what emerges with that invitation will be unwelcome. Some of it may make me uneasy. Some of it will be beautiful.

I want to be open to what is different. Not complacent, comfortable in the expected and the known. I want to risk change.

What will emerge?

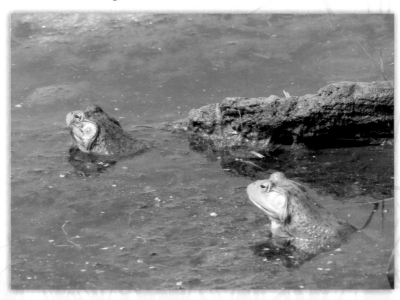

*Thomas Dean*

On the occasion of an Inipi ceremony at Prairiewoods Franciscan Spirituality Center, Hiawatha, Iowa:

*Midsummer brings*
*Water's abundance.*

*The rains enter the earth world*
*At the moment they resolve,*
*Filling the creeks in their full flow of self-emergence,*
*Filling the ponds with still depth, inviting marsh rise and frog song,*
*Feeding the soil, regenerating life itself.*

*On a midsummer night,*
*The water pourer decants earth's life-giving liquid*
*on the hot grandfather stones.*
*The transfigured spirit mist joins our breath in the womb of the earth.*
*From our sweat flow our mistakes, our anger, our sorrows.*
*From our breath we release our joy, our thanks, our truth.*
*Purification returns us to the source*
*And leads us into new wells of abundance.*
*We are all related.*

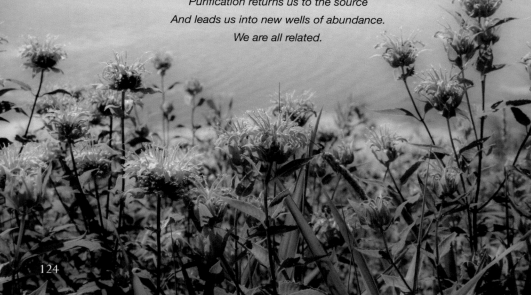

*The Hopi elder tells us,*
*"Know the river has its destination."*
*As we breathe, drink, fear, and grow from water's abundance,*
*We rejoin earth's beginnings,*
*And we trust it will take us to truth's ends.*

*Water's abundance is the source,*
*It is the path,*
*It is the end.*
*Our destiny is to join the river,*
*To trust it will take us to our authentic purpose.*

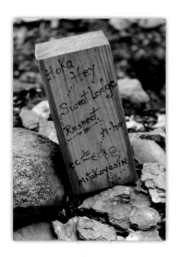

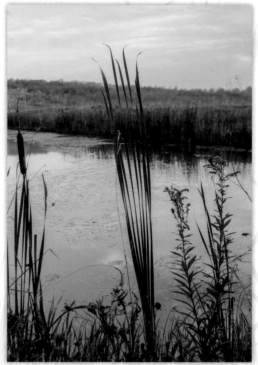

*conversation twenty-five*

# PERSISTENCE

*Cindy Crosby*

It's a ritual of autumn. The changing of our summer comforter to a heavy quilt, made for us by a friend. In the winter, when sleet taps against the window, I slip into bed and pull the quilt close under my chin. Admire the patchwork. Taupe, rust, emerald, peach. Grass-green and olive. Pearl. Oyster.

As he quilted, our friend incorporated the transient autumn colors of prairie grasses into the coverlet. I felt nestled into the prairie itself. Deep under. I might go dormant. Sleep for several months. Awaken to a cleansing fire in February and leaf out. Be fresher. Vibrant. Renewed.

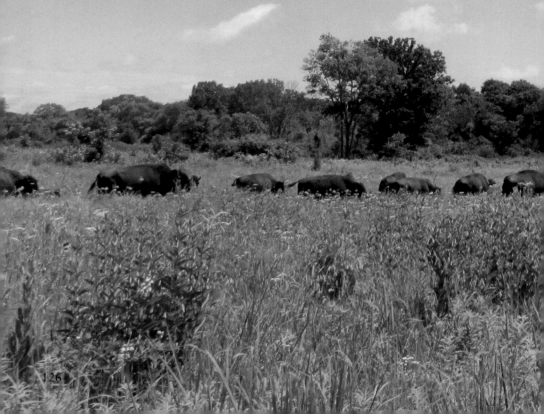

It's a heavy quilt, made from denims and corduroys, a quilt that—like the Midwestern prairies—looks resilient and ready to handle anything the future might throw at it. A quilt for the ages.

As I slipped off to sleep one night, I thought of the thousands of tiny stitches in this quilt and the prairie it reflects. The time and the care that one person put into one quilt. And the time and the care—all the "stitches" that have been put into the protection and repair of the grasslands that have been lost to us in the Midwest.

How will the grasslands "quilt" be patched back together?

We need the conservationist in the field who is bringing back the bison. *One stitch.*

We need the research student who is trying to understand why the bison make a difference to the upland sandpipers and the prairie vole and the dung beetle. *Stitch. Stitch. Stitch.*

The visitor who stumbles across a prairie and sees something of value. She isn't sure what she's looking at. But she can tell it is something special. So she takes a class, reads a book, or goes for a guided walk to learn a little bit more. *Stitch.*

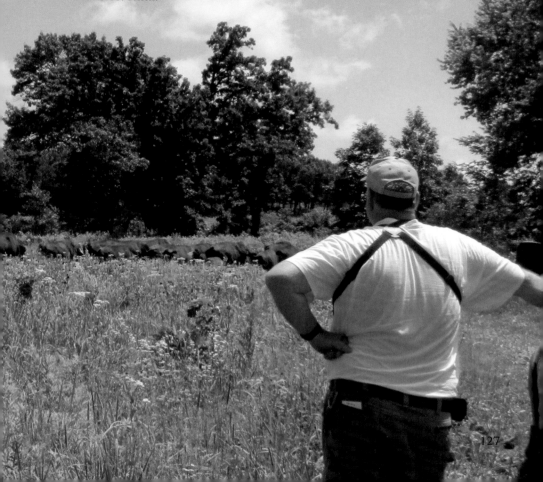

We need the steward who cares for the remnant where the bison are browsing and who reconstructs new prairie plantings close by. She knows these new plantings won't exactly replicate the old, but she hopes, *she hopes. . . .*

The activist at the state capitol who has ridden the bus, marched with a sign, and spent the day pleading the case of the natural world to the legislators. *Stitch.*

We need the poet who sees little bluestem, red and wet under November rains, rippling in the wind, and wrestles with just the right words to share what she sees on paper. *More stitches.*

Or the textile artist, the photographer, or the painter creating images that share prairie in ways that open doors of understanding to those who may not have experienced prairie before. *Stitch.*

The gardeners who make their backyards their painter's palettes. They plant prairie patches that swirl and glimmer with color and motion. A neighbor pauses. Asks a question. A spark is kindled. *Another stitch.*

Or people like my friend the quilter, who took up his needle and created something beautiful.

Each person who places each stitch—one carefully thought-out restoration, one painstakingly done research study on hands and knees in the cold and rain—each photograph, wall hanging, poem, book, song, painting, quilt—adds another stitch to the patches of the prairie patchwork quilt. Brings us closer to the beautiful whole of the Midwestern tallgrass that once was complete and now is lost.

Keep hoping. Keep stitching.

Persist.

Sweet dreams.

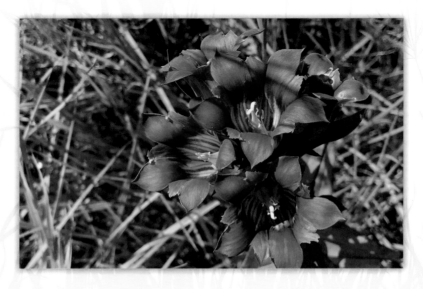

*Thomas Dean*

The essence of wildness—the self-regeneration of an ecosystem—is persistence. The native prairie knew how to persist. When our restorations do it, we can applaud some measure of success.

The essence of music—sound patterns that generate new sound patterns—is persistence. When a performance persists in sound variations, transformations, and returns that engage us, we applaud a successful composition.

Every spring, we rejoice when the shooting star and hoary puccoon make their showy emergence. The prairie persists! When the famous four notes of the opening of Beethoven's Fifth Symphony reemerge with blaring clarity at the first movement's climax, we thrill at the thematic return. The music persists!

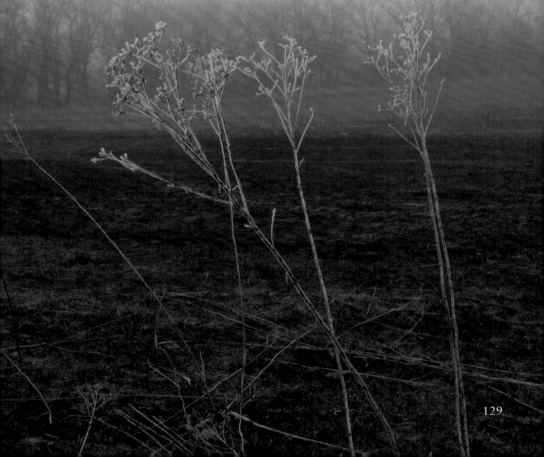

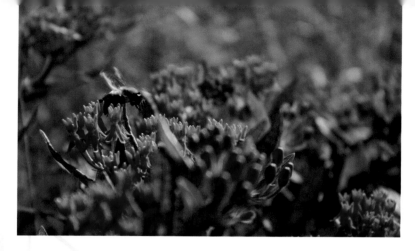

Yet the prairie's wildflowers and Beethoven's melodic motif are not the engines of persistence. They are the signs, the symbols, the capstones to an underlying structure that is much deeper and much more complex. Melody is crucial to harmonic music, but by itself, it is what we might sing in the shower or whistle while gardening. Wildflowers are the signs of vibrancy and life on the prairie, but by themselves, they please our eyes and maybe nostrils, and they attract our camera lenses (yes, and pollinators).

Harmonic and rhythmic variation are often the building blocks of persistence in Western classical music—that is, what infuses a piece with life and complexity beyond the statement of a melody. Melody sometimes undergirds those variations—the repetition of a *basso ostinato* upon which other layers of melody and harmony are laid, for example. The *basso ostinato* generates the composition and holds the piece together, but it's rarely what we sing in the shower. In much Eastern music as well, compositions often build their persistence on a melodic groundwork—the Indian *raga* or Javanese *balungan*, for example, upon which improvisations and elaborations demonstrate the skill and aesthetics we enjoy and applaud.

So what is the prairie's *raga* or *balungan*, its *basso ostinato* fueling its persistence if it's not the beauty of the spring and summer flowers we rejoice in? As with musical pieces, where the essential bass line may be buried by the harmonic, rhythmic, and other melodic complexities and beauties above it, the prairie's persistence lies deep in its soil.

As Wendell Berry says in *The Unsettling of America* ("The Use of Energy"), "The soil is the great connector of lives, the source and destination of all." The prairie's decomposition of organic matter is miraculous thanks to deep roots and fungal mats. Soil microbes play their industrious ground melody over and over again across time, creating carbon and nitrogen cycles (and so much more) that regenerate the beautiful persistent life above that we call "the prairie." In the soil, we don't see or hear the repeating foundational songs of microaggregates and macroaggregates, but we revel in the arias and *obbligatos* that are spiderwort, columbine, and prairie orchid.

Persistence lies below. Sing on your melodies of persistence, prairie, below your songs of beauty.

# TRUST

*Thomas Dean*

Without forethought or analysis, you instinctively know when you are home. You understand that unqualified love, safety, meaning, and nourishment—physical, emotional, spiritual—are there for you. Trust in home is our willingness to embrace this implicit knowledge. My trust in prairie as my home seems to have preceded my knowledge of prairie. I attribute that to prairie roots.

I grew up in an industrial city in northern Illinois. My childhood forays through the countryside—to go on vacation to Wisconsin, to visit relatives a few towns away, to make our way to Chicago to visit the Museum of Science and Industry—passed miles and miles of corn rather than bluestem. There literally were no prairies in my childhood, which I lived on land that had been entirely tallgrass only a century and a half before.

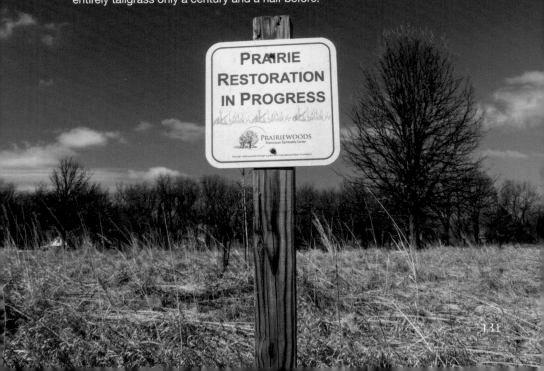

PRAIRIE
RESTORATION
IN PROGRESS

PRAIRIEWOODS
Franciscan Spirituality Center

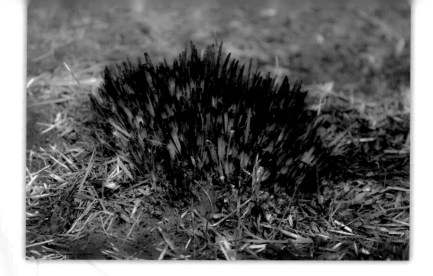

I consciously fell in love with the prairie when I learned more about it as an adult—what it had been, what remained of it, efforts to restore it. But that love had been latent since childhood. Growing up near the farm fields of Illinois, I saw plenty of wide horizons and open fields, and I identified with that essential flatland geography. But now having connected with prairie remnants and restorations, I know deep within me that, even as a child, I did not find my sense of home in cornfields. Yet I can't draw on childhood experience to compose love arias to the blooms of Culver's root and prairie smoke. I have to dig deeper. Without sideoats grama to tickle my feet or mountain mint to please my nose, my latent childhood love for the prairie—my trust in it as home—lay in its roots.

We trust that home—where we find shelter, sanctuary, and belonging—will always be there for us, even when we don't see it, even when we are far from it, indeed even if it no longer physically exists. We entrust ourselves to the roots of home that run deeper than we can fully perceive. Most of the mass of a prairie lies unseen underground, with roots growing twelve or more feet, holding water and holding soil, the life of the prairie. And despite the plowing, planting, and tilling of the past century and a half, even among the monocrop fields of corn and soybeans that comprise two-thirds of my adopted home of Iowa, native prairie roots lie still and deep yet today. At the end of the beautiful documentary *America's Lost Landscape: The Tallgrass Prairie*, anthropologist, writer, landscape architect, and Ioway tribal member Lance Foster says, "Prairie is alive. It may sleep, but underneath the invasive grasses, underneath the carved-up subdivisions, that land is still there. . . . The prairie, as long as there's one stem of grass somewhere, it'll come back."

My trust—my home—lies in prairie roots, and somehow that trust has been with me since I was born. I know those roots are there. I trust that they will be there when I most need them, and I trust that they will continue to break the surface as we bring our prairie home back into our lives.

## Cindy Crosby

As I get older, my memory is a dicey proposition. When I teach prairie ethnobotany, prairie wildflowers, and other natural history classes, I suddenly find myself fumbling for the scientific name to give my attentive students. Other times, I can't seem to do something as simple as pull the common name out of the proverbial hat. *Ummm . . . compass plant?* What dark vault of the mind did that name slip into where retrieval is questionable?

At least I can laugh about it. And trust that somewhere, deep in my memory, that information is still floating around somewhere.

I'm aware of the many sensory distractions of the suburbs where I live vying for space in what memory I do have available. Everywhere I turn, there is music playing—the coffee shop, the pharmacy, even the McDonald's drive-thru window where I grab some french fries (a guilty pleasure). The sounds of jets from three different airports are a constant soundtrack on one of the prairies I enjoy hiking, their contrails a reminder that no place is truly far from technology and civilization no matter how we label it a "natural area," or even "pristine wilderness."

In my backyard prairie patch, the scent of someone grilling hamburgers wafts on the breeze, or worse, the stink from a local sewage plant vies with the fragrance of prairie wildflowers. At Nachusa Grasslands, where I volunteer as a steward, the nuclear towers a few miles away are a constant distraction on the horizon.

The prairie is a mental oasis from all of this. I go and trust that nine times out of ten, I'll come away more clear-headed, thoughtful, centered. Yes, it has its own sensory overload, especially in the warmer months when pale purple coneflowers, Culver's root, and butterfly weed are jostling for attention; rampant birdsong orchestrates a warbled soundtrack; and the smells of wild bergamot and common milkweed fill the air.

Still. After more than two decades, the prairie offers respite. Clarity. Calm.

I reach the prairie and turn off my phone. Sit for a while. Observe. Walk a little bit. Sit some more. I can almost feel my mental muddle dissolve as I inhale the crisp air. Exhale some tension. Watch a bee buzzing around, looking for something to pollinate.

The deep, deep roots of the prairie plants—invisible, yet I know they are there—are anchors for me. I feel grounded, knowing what's under my feet. "What is essential is invisible to the eye," wrote Antoine de Saint-Exupéry, and so it is, isn't it?

After a baptism by fire each spring, the prairie seems obliterated. Destroyed. Ashes to ashes. And in a matter of weeks, we see it begin to grow and to write a new seasonal story.

I can point to times in my life when I felt as if nothing good would come from a terrible experience. Indeed, it is true that sometimes nothing good did come from it. And yet I began to write new chapters in my life. New stories. The prairie burn each season reminds me of this. It encourages me that resurrection from the darkest night of the soul is possible.

On the newly burned prairie, I trust that growth is just around the corner. I remember what each season before has brought, and I trust in the cycle of the seasons. I believe in what I don't see because I know what the patterns are. A burned landscape has potential for so much more than meets the eye. I trust the patterns will continue—a cycle of growth, renewal, abundance, slowing down, rest.

The tallgrass doesn't solve my problems. But it does help give me perspective.

It helps me trust in something more.

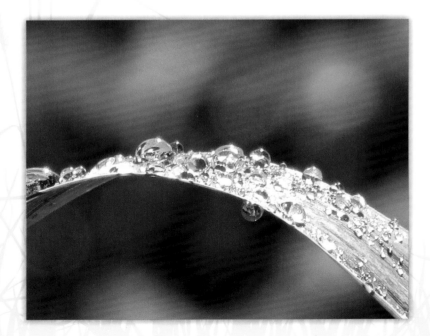

# ENDNOTES

**INTRODUCTION**

**Cindy Crosby**

The Nature Conservancy: https://support.nature.org/site/Advocacy?cmd=display&page=UserAction&id=150

John T. Price, Introduction, *The Tallgrass Prairie Reader* (Iowa City, IA: University of Iowa Press, 2014), xix.

Gerould Wilhelm & Laura Rericha, *Flora of the Chicago Region: A Floristic and Ecological Synthesis* (Indianapolis, IN: Indiana Academy of Science, 2017), 5.

**CONVERSATION 1: PATH**

**Thomas Dean**

This essay is in part an homage to Paul Gruchow's "What the Prairie Teaches Us," in *Grass Roots: The Universe of Home* (Minneapolis, MN: Milkweed Editions, 1995), 77–82.

**CONVERSATION 2: POSSIBILITIES**

**Cindy Crosby**

First published in a slightly different format as part of a longer essay, "Divine Hours Spent Hiking with God," in "Traveling Well," ed. Robert B. Kruschwitz, *Christian Reflection: A Series in Faith and Ethics* (Institute for Faith and Learning, Baylor University), 60 (2016): 28–37. This material is used with permission of the publisher.

"The Journey," Mary Oliver, in *New and Selected Poems* (Boston: Beacon Press, 1993), 114.

**CONVERSATION 3: WORDS**

**Cindy Crosby**

This essay originally appeared in a different form in Cindy Crosby's *Tuesdays in the Tallgrass* blog, https://tuesdaysinthetallgrass.wordpress.com.

The Nature Conservancy: https://www.nature.org/ourinitiatives/urgentissues/land-conservation/grasslands/index.htm.

**Thomas Dean**

Hamlin Garland, *Boy Life on the Prairie* (Lincoln, NE: Bison Books/University of Nebraska Press, 1961).

**CONVERSATION 4: HOME**

**Cindy Crosby**

This essay originally appeared in a slightly different form in Cindy Crosby's *Tuesdays in the Tallgrass* blog, https://tuesdaysinthetallgrass.wordpress.com.

**CONVERSATION 5: LOSS**

Cindy Crosby

This essay originally appeared in a slightly different form in Cindy Crosby's *Tuesdays in the Tallgrass* blog, https://tuesdaysinthetallgrass.wordpress.com.

**CONVERSATION 6: HEALING**

**Cindy Crosby**

This essay originally appeared in a slightly different form in Cindy Crosby's *Tuesdays in the Tallgrass* blog, https://tuesdaysinthetallgrass.wordpress.com.

Rainer Maria Rilke, *The Duino Elegies (Ninth)*. This translation is from https://www.poetrysociety.org/psa/poetry/crossroads/own_words/Rainer_Maria_Rilke/.

Dean Roosa and Sy Runkel, *Wildflowers of the Tallgrass Prairie: The Upper Midwest* (Ames, IA: Iowa State University Press 1989), 161.

David E. Moerman, *Native American Ethnobotany* (Portland, OR: Timber Press, 1998), 205–06.

**Thomas Dean**

Wendell Berry, "Health Is Membership," in *Another Turn of the Crank* (Washington, DC: Counterpoint, 1995), 86–109.

**CONVERSATION 7: REMNANT**

**Thomas Dean**

The Aldo Leopold Foundation is carefully harvesting a number of "Leopold" pines for conservation purposes. The Leopold family planted thousands of pines on their land near the Wisconsin River in their restoration efforts, which are now mature. Some are being carefully harvested for the health of the land.

**Cindy Crosby**

Gerould Wilhelm and Laura Rericha, *Flora of the Chicago Region: A Floristic and Eco-*

*logical Synthesis* (Indianapolis, IN: Indiana Academy of Science, 2017), 4–5.

### Conversation 9: LISTENING

**Cindy Crosby**

First published in a slightly different format as part of a longer essay, "Divine Hours Spent Hiking with God," in *Traveling Well*, Christian Reflection: A Series in Faith and Ethics (Institute for Faith and Learning, Baylor University), ed. Robert B. Kruschwitz, 60 (2016): 28–37. This material is used with permission of the publisher.

**Thomas Dean**

The Belden Lane quotation was provided in materials from Lane's retreat entitled "The Great Conversation: Nature and the Care of the Soul" at Prairiewoods Franciscan Spirituality Center, Hiawatha, Iowa, March 16–18, 2018.

Linda Hogan, "A Different Yield," in *Dwellings: A Spiritual History of the Living World* (New York: W. W. Norton, 1995), 47–62.

### Conversation 10: STILLNESS

**Thomas Dean**

Wendell Berry, "The Peace of Wild Things," *Openings: Poems* (New York: Harcourt, Brace & World, 1968), 30.

### Conversation 11: PATIENCE

**Cindy Crosby**

This essay originally appeared in a slightly different form in Cindy Crosby's *Tuesdays in the Tallgrass* blog, https://tuesdaysinthetallgrass.wordpress.com.

**Thomas Dean**

An earlier version of this essay appeared under the title "Unframing Nature" in *Little Village* (Iowa City, IA), May 4, 2016, 6–7.

Richard Louv, *The Nature Principle: Reconnecting with Life in a Virtual Age* (Chapel Hill, NC: Algonquin Books, 2012).

### Conversation 12: JOY

**Cindy Crosby**

This essay originally appeared in a slightly different form in Cindy Crosby's *Tuesdays in the Tallgrass* blog, https://tuesdaysinthetallgrass.wordpress.com.

David Moerman, *Native American Ethnobotany* (Portland, OR: Timber Press, 1998), 312.

### Conversation 13: SURPRISE

**Cindy Crosby**

This essay originally appeared in a slightly different form in Cindy Crosby's *Tuesdays in the Tallgrass* blog, https://tuesdaysinthetallgrass.wordpress.com.

Jack Sanders, *The Secrets of Wildflowers* (Guilford, CT: Lyons Press–Rowman & Littlefield, 2014), 3–6.

### Conversation 14: WONDER

**Cindy Crosby**

This essay originally appeared in a slightly different form in Cindy Crosby's *Tuesdays in the Tallgrass* blog, https://tuesdaysinthetallgrass.wordpress.com.

Sigurd Olson, *Listening Point* (New York: Alfred A. Knopf, 1980), 2.

Mary Oliver, "Wild Geese," in *New and Selected Poems* (Boston: Beacon Press, 1993), 110.

**Thomas Dean**

Rachel Carson, *The Sense of Wonder: A Celebration of Nature for Parents and Children* (New York: Harper Perennial, 1956, 2017).

### Conversation 15: MAJESTY

**Cindy Crosby**

This essay originally appeared in a slightly different form in Cindy Crosby's *Tuesdays in the Tallgrass* blog, https://tuesdaysinthetallgrass.wordpress.com.

Aldo Leopold, *Round River*, ed. Luna B. Leopold (New York: Oxford University Press, 1953), 147.

### Conversation 16: DIVERSITY

**Cindy Crosby**

First published in a slightly different format as part of a longer essay, "Divine Hours Spent Hiking with God," in *Traveling Well*, Christian Reflection: A Series in Faith and Ethics (Institute for Faith and Learning, Baylor University), ed. Robert B. Kruschwitz, 60 (2016): 28–37. This material is used with permission of the publisher.

**Thomas Dean**

Paul Gruchow, "What the Prairie Teaches Us," in *Grass Roots: The Universe of Home* (Minneapolis, MN: Milkweed Editions, 1995), 77–82.

## CONVERSATION 17: DESIGN

**Thomas Dean**

The original version of this poem was composed at a session of the "Regenerative Leadership for the Creative Corridor" series of retreats conducted by the Center for Regenerative Society, led by Benjamin Webb and Stephanie Clohesy, held at Prairiewoods Franciscan Spirituality Center, Hiawatha, Iowa, January 2015.

**Cindy Crosby**

Georgia O'Keeffe, quoted in Laurie Lisle, *Portrait of an Artist: A Biography of Georgia O'Keeffe* (New York: Washington Square Press, 1997), 61.

W. John Hayden, "Bloodroot Pollination: Bet-Hedging in Uncertain Times," *Bulletin of the Virginia Native Plant Society* (February 2005): 5–6.

## CONVERSATION 19: DIRECTION

**Thomas Dean**

The original version of this essay was composed for a workshop led by Mary Swander called "A Writer's Ecology: Reading and Writing as Transformation" at Prairiewoods Franciscan Spirituality Center, Hiawatha, Iowa, July 25–27, 2017.

**Cindy Crosby**

This poem first appeared in a slightly different form in www.APrairieJournal. All rights retained by the author.

## CONVERSATION 20: MYSTERY

**Cindy Crosby**

This essay originally appeared in a slightly different form in Cindy Crosby's *Tuesdays in the Tallgrass* blog, https://tuesdaysin-thetallgrass.wordpress.com.

The quotation from Agatha Christie is the subtitle of her book *The Mysterious Affair at Styles: Instinct is a Marvelous Thing. It Can Neither be Explained or Ignored* (London: John Lane, 1920).

For more information and articles that helped inform this essay, please visit and support the Xerces Society at www.xerces.org.

## CONVERSATION 21: DEPTH

**Cindy Crosby**

A version of this essay titled "Fieldwork: More than Data" appeared on the blog *Dispatches from the Field*, March 7, 2018, https://dispatchesfromthefield1.word-press.com/2018/03/07/fieldwork-more-than-data/.

## CONVERSATION 22: SHADOW

**Thomas Dean**

David Whyte, "Shadow," from *Consolations: The Solace, Nourishment and Underlying Meaning of Everyday Words* (Langley, WA: Many Rivers Press, 2015), 205–08.

**Cindy Crosby**

This essay originally appeared in a slightly different form in Cindy Crosby's *Tuesdays in the Tallgrass* blog, https://tuesdaysin-thetallgrass.wordpress.com.

Martin Luther King, Jr., quotation slightly paraphrased from "The Dimensions of a Complete Life," *The Papers of Martin Luther King, Jr.,* ed. Clayborne Carson, Tenisha Hart Armstrong, Adrienne Clay, Susan Carson, and Kieran Taylor, vol. 5, *Threshold of a New Decade, January 1959–December 1960* (Berkeley: University of California Press, 2005), 578.

## CONVERSATION 23: TRANSITIONS

**Cindy Crosby**

This essay originally appeared in a slightly different form in Cindy Crosby's *Tuesdays in the Tallgrass* blog, https://tuesdaysin-thetallgrass.wordpress.com.

**Thomas Dean**

The original version of this poem was composed at a session of the "Regenerative Leadership for the Creative Corridor" series of retreats conducted by the Center for Regenerative Society, led by Benjamin Webb and Stephanie Clohesy, held at Prairiewoods Franciscan Spirituality Center, Hiawatha, Iowa, April 2015.

## CONVERSATION 24: CHANGE

**Cindy Crosby**

First published in a slightly different format as part of a longer essay, "Divine Hours Spent Hiking with God," in *Traveling Well*, Christian Reflection: A Series in Faith and Ethics (Institute for Faith and Learning, Baylor University), ed. Robert

B. Kruschwitz, 60 (2016): 28–37. This material is used with permission of the publisher.

**Thomas Dean**

The original version of this poem was composed at a session of the "Regenerative Leadership for the Creative Corridor" series of retreats conducted by the Center for Regenerative Society, led by Benjamin Webb and Stephanie Clohesy, held at Prairiewoods Franciscan Spirituality Center, Hiawatha, Iowa, June 2015.

## CONVERSATION 25: PERSISTENCE

**Cindy Crosby**

This essay originally appeared in a slightly different form in Cindy Crosby's *Tuesdays in the Tallgrass* blog, https://tuesdaysin-thetallgrass.wordpress.com.

With thanks to Louise Erdrich for her essay "Big Grass," which helped inspire part of this conversation, included in *The Tallgrass Prairie Reader*, ed. John T. Price (Iowa City, IA: University of Iowa Press, 2014), 225–30.

**Thomas Dean**

Wendell Berry, "The Use of Energy," in *The Unsettling of America: Culture and Agriculture* (San Francisco: Sierra Club Books, 1977), 81–95.

## CONVERSATION 26: TRUST

**Thomas Dean**

Essential concepts and a few sentences of this essay first appeared in my essay "Prairie Home," *Rootstalk*, 1 (2015): 8–12.

*America's Lost Landscape: The Tallgrass Prairie*, directed by David O'Shields, produced by David O'Shields and Daryl Smith, Bullfrog Films, 2005.

**Cindy Crosby**

Antoine de Saint-Exupéry, chap. 21, *The Little Prince* (1943), in *Oxford Essential Quotations*, 4th ed., ed. Susan Ratcliffe (New York: Oxford University Press, 2106), online at oxfordreference.com/view/10.1093/acref/9780191826719.001.0001/q-oro-ed4-00009075.

# PHOTO CREDITS

Cover, top: Schulenberg Prairie, The Morton Arboretum, Lisle, IL. *Cindy Crosby*

Cover, bottom: Cup plant (*Silphium perfoliatum*), Herbert Hoover National Historic Site Tallgrass Prairie, West Branch, IA. *Thomas Dean*

Title page, top: Nachusa Grasslands, Franklin Grove, IL. *Cindy Crosby*

Title page, bottom: Wild bergamot (*Monarda fistulosa*), Prairiewoods Franciscan Spirituality Center, Hiawatha, IA. *Thomas Dean*

P. 9: Neal Smith National Wildlife Refuge, Prairie City, IA. *Thomas Dean*

Pp. 10–11: Herbert Hoover National Historic Site Tallgrass Prairie, West Branch, IA. *Thomas Dean*

P. 11, inset: Neal Smith National Wildlife Refuge, Prairie City, IA. *Thomas Dean*

Pp. 12–13: Bison (*Bison bison*), Nachusa Grasslands, Franklin Grove, IL. *Cindy Crosby*

P. 13, inset: Indian grass (*Sorghastrum nutans*), Gabis Arboretum at Purdue

Northwest, Valparaiso, IN. *Cindy Crosby*

P. 14: Prescribed burn, Schulenberg Prairie, The Morton Arboretum, Lisle, IL. *Cindy Crosby*

P. 15: Pasque flowers (*Potentilla patens*), Nachusa Grasslands, Franklin Grove, IL. *Cindy Crosby*

Pp. 16–17: Neal Smith National Wildlife Refuge, Prairie City, IA. *Thomas Dean*

P. 16, inset: Swamp white oak (*Quercus bicolor*) leaf, Prairiewoods Franciscan Spirituality Center, Hiawatha, IA. *Thomas Dean*

P. 17, inset: White wild indigo (*Baptisa alba macrophylla*), F. W. Kent Park, Johnson County Conservation, Oxford, IA. *Thomas Dean*

Pp. 18–19: Jeff Crosby reading at Nachusa Grasslands, Franklin Grove, IL. *Cindy Crosby*

P. 19: Street sign, Chana, IL. *Cindy Crosby*

Pp. 20–21: Neal Smith National Wildlife Refuge, Prairie City, IA. *Thomas Dean*

Pp. 22–23: Oak savanna, Prairiewoods Franciscan Spirituality Center, Hiawatha, IA. *Thomas Dean*

P. 23, inset: Remnant savanna bur oak (*Quercus macrocarpa*), Neal Smith National Wildlife Refuge, Prairie City, IA. *Thomas Dean*

P. 24: Oak savanna, Herbert Hoover National Historic Site Tallgrass Prairie, West Branch, IA. *Thomas Dean*

P. 25: Chinese mantis (*Tenodera sinensis*) egg case, Orland Grasslands, Orland Park, IL. *Cindy Crosby*

Pp. 26–27: Nachusa Grasslands, Franklin Grove, IL. *Cindy Crosby*

P. 29: Pale purple coneflower (*Echinacea pallida*), Schulenberg Prairie, The Morton Arboretum, Lisle, IL. *Cindy Crosby*

P. 30, inset: Bird's nest, Nachusa Grasslands, Franklin Grove, IL. *Cindy Crosby*

Pp. 30–31: Belmont Prairie, Downers Grove, IL. *Cindy Crosby*

P. 32: Ohio spiderwort (*Tradescantia ohiensis*), Rochester Cemetery, Cedar County, IA. *Thomas Dean*

P. 33: Rochester Cemetery, Cedar County, IA. *Thomas Dean*

P. 34: Rochester Cemetery, Cedar County, IA. *Thomas Dean*

P. 35: Pale purple coneflower (*Echinacea pallida*), Schulenberg Prairie, The Morton Arboretum, Lisle, IL. *Cindy Crosby*

P. 36, inset: Pale purple coneflower (*Echinacea allida*) with fasciation, Belmont Prairie, Downers Grove, IL. *Cindy Crosby*

Pp. 36–37: White wild indigo (*Baptisia alba macrophylla*) with pale purple coneflowers (*Echinacea pallida*) and other wildflowers, Nachusa Grasslands, Franklin Grove, IL. *Cindy Crosby*

Pp. 38–39: Wild bergamot (*Monarda fistulosa*), Prairiewoods Franciscan Spirituality Center, Hiawatha, IA. *Thomas Dean*

P. 40: Culver's root (*Veronicastrum virginicum*) and rattlesnake master (*Eryngium yuccifolium*), Prairiewoods Franciscan Spirituality Center, Hiawatha, IA. *Thomas Dean*

P. 41: Wild columbine (*Aquilegia canadensis*), Rochester Cemetery, Cedar County, IA. *Thomas Dean*

Pp. 42–43: Hitchcock Nature Center, Pottawattamie County Conservation, Loess Hills, Honey Creek, IA. *Thomas Dean*

P. 44: Bronze copper butterfly (*Lycaena hyllus*), Nachusa Grasslands, Franklin Grove, IL. *Cindy Crosby*

P. 45: Familiar bluet damselfly (*Enallagma civile*), Nachusa Grasslands, Franklin Grove, IL. *Cindy Crosby*

Pp. 46–47: Tony Buono explores the Schulenberg Prairie, The Morton Arboretum, Lisle, IL. *Cindy Crosby*

P. 48: White wild indigo (*Baptisia alba macrophylla*) with volunteer Kath Thomas weeding, Schulenberg Prairie, The Morton Arboretum, Lisle, IL. *Cindy Crosby*

P. 49: Leopold Shack prairie, Aldo Leopold Foundation, Columbia County, WI. *Thomas Dean*

P. 50: Poppy mallow (*Callirhoe triangulata*), Leopold Shack prairie, Aldo Leopold Foundation, Columbia County, WI. *Thomas Dean*

P. 51: Metalwork at International Crane Foundation prairie, Baraboo, WI. *Cindy Crosby*

Pp. 52–53: Sandhill cranes (*Antigone canadensis*) migrating, Jasper-Pulaski Fish & Wildlife Area, Medaryville, IN. *Cindy Crosby*

P. 54: Old and new grasses, Prairiewoods Franciscan Spirituality Center, Hiawatha, IA. *Thomas Dean*

P. 55: Common milkweed (*Asclepias syriaca*) with monarch (*Danaus plexippus*) caterpillar, Herbert Hoover National Historic Site Tallgrass Prairie, West Branch, IA. *Thomas Dean*

Pp. 56–57: Cattails (*Typhus latifolia*), Waterworks Prairie Park, Iowa City, IA. *Thomas Dean*

P. 58: Big bluestem (*Andropogon gerardii*), F. W. Kent Park, Johnson County Conservation, Oxford, IA. *Thomas Dean*

P. 59: Fermilab Natural Areas prairie, Fermilab National Accelerator Laboratory, Batavia, IL. *Cindy Crosby*

P. 60: Fame Flower Knob, Nachusa Grasslands, Franklin Grove, IL. *Cindy Crosby*

P. 61: Bee on pasture thistle (*Cirsium discolor*), Schulenberg Prairie, The Morton Arboretum, Lisle, IL. *Cindy Crosby*

P. 62: Harvesting seed at Midewin National Tallgrass Prairie, Wilmington, IL. *Cindy Crosby*

P. 63: Neal Smith National Wildlife Refuge, Prairie City, IA. *Thomas Dean*

Pp. 64–65: Neal Smith National Wildlife Refuge, Prairie City, IA. *Thomas Dean*

P. 65, inset: Emerging plant, Prairiewoods Franciscan Spirituality Center, Hiawatha, IA. *Thomas Dean*

P. 67: Hickory Hill Park, Iowa City, IA. *Thomas Dean*

P. 68: Cardinal flower (*Lobelia cardinalis*) and swamp milkweed (*Asclepius incarnata*), Nomia Meadows Farm prairie and wetlands, Franklin Grove, IL. *Cindy Crosby*

P. 69: Eastern black tiger swallowtail butterfly (*Papilio polyxenes asterius*) on gray-headed coneflower (*Ratibida pinnata*), Nachusa Grasslands, Franklin Grove, IL. *Cindy Crosby*

P. 70: Cardinal flower (*Lobelia cardinalis*), Nomia Meadows Farm prairie and wetlands, Franklin Grove, IL. *Cindy Crosby*

P. 71: Pale purple coneflower (*Echinacea pallida*), F. W. Kent Park, Johnson County Conservation, Oxford, IA. *Thomas Dean*

Pp. 72–74: Cup plants (*Silphium perfoliatum*), Herbert Hoover National Historic Site Tallgrass Prairie, West Branch, IA. *Thomas Dean*

P. 73, inset: American goldfinch (*Spinus tristis*), Herbert Hoover National Historic Site Tallgrass Prairie, West Branch, IA. *Thomas Dean*

P. 74: Big bluestem (*Andropogon gerardii*), Herbert Hoover National Historic Site Tallgrass Prairie, West Branch, IA. *Thomas Dean*

P. 75: Horsetail (*Equisetum arvense*), Neal Smith National Wildlife Refuge, Prairie City, IA. *Thomas Dean*

P. 76: Feather, Conard Environmental Research Area, Grinnell College, Grinnell, IA. *Thomas Dean*

P. 77: Pasque flowers (*Pulsatilla patens*), Schulenberg Prairie, The Morton Arboretum, Lisle, IL. *Cindy Crosby*

P. 78: Harbinger-of-spring (*Erigenia bulbosa*), Schulenberg Prairie savanna, The Morton Arboretum, Lisle, IL. *Cindy Crosby*

P. 79: Canada geese (*Branta canadensis*), Schulenberg Prairie, The Morton Arboretum, Lisle, IL. *Cindy Crosby*

P. 80: White wild indigo (*Baptisia alba macrophylla*), Schulenberg Prairie, The Morton Arboretum, Lisle, IL. *Cindy Crosby*

P. 81: Shooting star (*Dodecatheon meadia*), F. W. Kent Park, Johnson County Conservation, Oxford, IA. *Thomas Dean*

P. 82: Shooting star (*Dodecatheon meadia*), F. W. Kent Park, Johnson County Conservation, Oxford, IA. *Thomas Dean*

P. 83: Bison (*Bison bison*), Neal Smith National Wildlife Refuge, Prairie City, IA. *Thomas Dean*

P. 84: Herbert Hoover National Historic Site Tallgrass Prairie, West Branch, IA. *Thomas Dean*

P. 85: Bison (*Bison bison*), Nachusa Grasslands, Franklin Grove, IL. *Cindy Crosby*

P. 86: White lady's slipper orchid (*Cypripedium candidum*), Schulenberg Prairie, The Morton Arboretum, Lisle, IL. *Cindy Crosby*

P. 87: Ebony jewelwing damselfly (*Calopteryx maculata*) with unknown spider, Willoway Brook, Schulenberg Prairie, The Morton Arboretum, Lisle, IL. *Cindy Crosby*

Pp. 88–89: Nachusa Grasslands, Franklin Grove, IL. *Cindy Crosby*

Pp. 90–91: Herbert Hoover National Historic Site Tallgrass Prairie, West Branch, IA. *Thomas Dean*

P. 92: Prairiewoods Franciscan Spirituality Center, Hiawatha, IA. *Thomas Dean*

P. 93: Monarchs (*Danaus plexippus*) nectaring on stiff goldenrod (*Oligoneuron rigidum*), Kankakee Sands, Morocco, IN. *Cindy Crosby*

P. 94: Black-eyed Susan (*Rudbeckia hirta*) seedhead, Herbert Hoover National Historic Site Tallgrass Prairie, West Branch, IA. *Thomas Dean*

P. 95: Bloodroot (*Sanguinaria canadensis*), Schulenberg Prairie savanna, The Morton Arboretum, Lisle, IL. *Cindy Crosby*

P. 96: Bee on white wild indigo (*Baptisia alba macrophylla*), Schulenberg Prairie, The Morton Arboretum, Lisle, IL. *Cindy Crosby*

P. 97: Half-moon, Herbert Hoover National Historic Site Tallgrass Prairie, West Branch, IA. *Thomas Dean*

P. 98: Road to Thelma Carpenter Prairie Unit, Nachusa Grasslands, Franklin Grove, IL. *Cindy Crosby*

P. 99 Little bluestem (*Schizachyrium scoparium*), Wolf Road Prairie Preserve, Westchester, IL. *Cindy Crosby*

P. 99: White vervain (*Verbena urticifolia*), Schulenberg Prairie Savanna, The Morton Arboretum, Lisle, IL. *Cindy Crosby*

Pp. 100–101: Compass plants (*Silphium laciniatum*), Conard Environmental Research Area, Grinnell College, Grinnell, IA. *Thomas Dean*

P. 102: Belmont Prairie, Downers Grove, IL. *Cindy Crosby*

P. 102, inset, top: Compass plant (*Silphium laciniatum*), Belmont Prairie, Downers Grove, IL. *Cindy Crosby*

P. 102, inset, bottom: Compass plant (*Silphium laciniatum*), Schulenberg Prairie, The Morton Arboretum, Lisle, IL. *Cindy Crosby*

P. 104: Canada wild rye (*Elymus canadensis*), Prairiewoods Franciscan Spirituality Center, Hiawatha, IA. *Thomas Dean*

P. 105, top: Big bluestem (*Andropogon gerardii*) after rain, Prairiewoods Franciscan Spirituality Center, Hiawatha, IA. *Thomas Dean*

P. 105, bottom: Big bluestem (*Andropogon gerardii*), Hickory Hill Park, Iowa City, IA. *Thomas Dean*

P. 106: Twelve-spotted skimmer dragonfly (*Libellula pulchella*) on purple prairie clover (*Dalea purpurea*), Schulenberg Prairie, The Morton Arboretum, Lisle, IL. *Cindy Crosby*

P. 107: Calico pennant dragonfly (*Celithemis elisa*), Schulenberg Prairie, The Morton Arboretum, Lisle, IL. *Cindy Crosby*

P. 108: Rabbit track, Herbert Hoover National Historic Site Tallgrass Prairie, West Branch, IA. *Thomas Dean*

P. 109: Prairie dock (*Silphium terebinthinaceum*) leaf, Herbert Hoover National Historic Site Tallgrass Prairie, West Branch, IA. *Thomas Dean*

Pp. 110–111: Nachusa Grasslands, Franklin Grove, IL. *Cindy Crosby*

P. 111, inset: Non-native Queen Anne's lace (*Daucus carota*), Afton Preserve Prairie, DeKalb County Forest Preserve, Malta, IL. *Cindy Crosby*

Pp. 112–113: Herbert Hoover National Historic Site Tallgrass Prairie, West Branch, IA. *Thomas Dean*

P. 113, inset: Prairie dock (*Silphium terebinthinaceum*) leaf, Herbert Hoover National Historic Site Tallgrass Prairie, West Branch, IA. *Thomas Dean*

P. 114: Feather, Schulenberg Prairie, The Morton Arboretum, Lisle, IL. *Cindy Crosby*

P. 115: Switchgrass (*Panicum virgatum*), Prairiewoods Franciscan Spirituality Center, Hiawatha, IA. *Cindy Crosby*

P. 117: Hidden Lake Forest Preserve, Forest Preserve District of DuPage County, Downers Grove, IL. *Cindy Crosby*

P. 118: Bridge over Willoway Brook, Schulenberg Prairie, The Morton Arboretum, Lisle, IL. *Cindy Crosby*

P. 119: Willoway Brook, Schulenberg Prairie, The Morton Arboretum, Lisle, IL. *Cindy Crosby*

P. 120: Prairiewoods Franciscan Spirituality Center, Hiawatha, IA. *Thomas Dean*

P. 120, inset: Conard Environmental Research Area, Grinnell College, Grinnell, IA. *Thomas Dean*

P. 122: Prairie wetlands, Nachusa Grasslands, Franklin Grove, IL. *Cindy Crosby*

P. 123: American bullfrogs (*Lithobates catesbeianus*), Nachusa Grasslands, Franklin Grove, IL. *Cindy Crosby*

P. 124: Wild bergamot (*Monarda fistulosa*), Conard Environmental Research Area, Grinnell College, Grinnell, IA. *Thomas Dean*

P. 125: Sweat lodge, Prairiewoods Franciscan Spirituality Center, Hiawatha, IA. *Thomas Dean*

P. 125: Cattails (*Typhus latifolia*), Solstead Retreat and Learning Center, Iowa County, IA. *Thomas Dean*

Pp. 126–127: Prairie steward John Heneghan watches bison (*Bison bison*) herd, Nachusa Grasslands, Franklin Grove, IL. *Cindy Crosby*

P. 128: Prairie gentians (*Gentiana puberulenta*), Schulenberg Prairie, The Morton Arboretum, Lisle, IL. *Cindy Crosby*

Page 129: Prairie after controlled burn, Prairiewoods Franciscan Spirituality Center, Hiawatha, IA. *Thomas Dean*

P. 130: Butterfly milkweed (*Asclepias tuberosa*), Neal Smith National Wildlife Refuge, Prairie City, IA. *Thomas Dean*

P. 131: Prairiewoods Franciscan Spirituality Center, Hiawatha, IA. *Thomas Dean*

P. 132: Prairie dropseed (*Sporobolus heterolepis*) after controlled burn, Prairiewoods Franciscan Spirituality Center, Hiawatha, IA. *Thomas Dean*

P. 133: Willoway Brook, Schulenberg Prairie, The Morton Arboretum, Lisle, IL. *Cindy Crosby*

P. 134: Clear Creek, Nachusa Grasslands, Franklin Grove, IL. *Cindy Crosby*

Back cover: top: Trail through the Tallgrass Prairie National Preserve, Strong City, KS. *Cindy Crosby*

Back cover, bottom: Cup plants (*Silphium perfoliatum*), Herbert Hoover National Historic Site Tallgrass Prairie, West Branch, IA. *Thomas Dean*

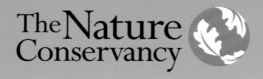

# The Nature Conservancy

Founded in 1951, The Nature Conservancy works in all 50 U.S. states and more than 70 countries. We address the most critical conservation issues for nature and people including climate change, food and water security, urban conservation and land and water protection.

Nature.org/Illinois

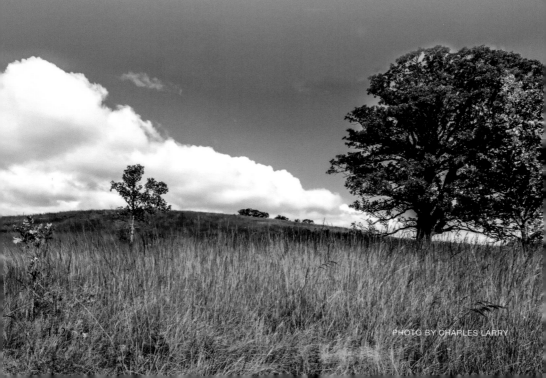

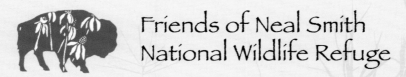

# Friends of Neal Smith National Wildlife Refuge

**THE FRIENDS OF NEAL SMITH NATIONAL WILDLIFE REFUGE** was founded in 1993 as a self-sustaining 501(c)3 non-profit organization. An all-volunteer group, the Friends promote public awareness of the Refuge and participation in the learning and growing that occur every day.

**WE PROVIDE** funding for projects and events beyond the reach of federally appropriated dollars. This includes funding for school field trips, internships, educational programs, seed purchases and land acquisitions to name a few. The Friends also operate the Prairie Point Nature Store in the Visitors Center with all proceeds supporting the Refuge.

**CONTACT INFORMATION:**
515-994-2918 • P.O. Box 114, Prairie City, IA 50228
Website: www.tallgrass.org • Email: buffalo@tallgrass.org

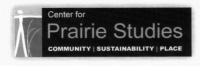

**The Center for Prairie Studies** promotes Grinnell College's location as a teaching and learning resource with special attention to themes of community, sustainability, and place. The Center's diverse programs encourage the exploration of links between the local and the global in this particular setting: the human place in nature, rural and urban dynamics, migration, food and agriculture, the politics and economics of local communities, and artistic responses to place.

https://www.grinnell.edu/academics/centers-programs/prairie-studies

**The Tallgrass Prairie Center** restores native vegetation for the benefit of society and environment through research, education, and technology.

**Contact information:**
Tallgrass Prairie Center
The University of Northern Iowa
2412 West 27th Street
Cedar Falls, Iowa 50614-0294
https://tallgrassprairiecenter.org/

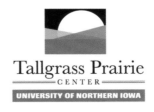

# ACKNOWLEDGMENTS

From Tom and Cindy—

We would like to thank our collaborative team: our incredibly supportive and intrepid publisher, Steve Semken of Ice Cube Press, and our tremendous designer, Cindy Kiple, who has brought our vision to reality in ways that have far exceeded our own powers and imagination. We also would like to enthusiastically thank our organizational supporters, whose generous contributions have made possible the publication of a book with color photographs, an increasing rarity today: the Nature Conservancy Illinois, Friends of the Neal Smith National Wildlife Refuge, the Center for Prairie Studies at Grinnell College, and the Tallgrass Prairie Center at the University of Northern Iowa. Their steadfast work is one of the reasons we have tallgrass prairie today.

From Tom—

My deepest appreciation goes to my highly talented (and patient) co-creator, Cindy Crosby, who was brave and bold enough to embark on this different type of "conversation" project. I would also like to humbly thank some remarkable teachers and organizations who inspired me during the creation of this book. My learning and work with them, in multiple ways, appear in *Tallgrass Conversations*: Mary Swander and her "A Writer's Ecology" retreat at Prairiewoods Franciscan Spirituality Center in Hiawatha, Iowa; Belden Lane and his "The Great Conversation: Nature and the Care of the Soul" retreat, also at Prairiewoods; and Kimberly Blaeser and her "Wisdom Sits in Places: Creative Writing from the Natural World" workshop at the Aldo Leopold Center in Baraboo, Wisconsin. You will also see in this book the significant influence on me of the work of Aldo Leopold, as well as that of Wendell Berry and David Whyte. My work on this book also rests on—in explicit and implicit ways—the profound influence of Paul Gruchow, whom I was fortunate to know as a friend and mentor before he left this world. And, of course, I am always grateful for the love, support, and patience of my family—Susan, Nathaniel, and Sylvia—as creating a book is always exhilarating but never easy.

From Cindy—

This book would not have happened without the thoughtful and talented Tom Dean, who asked, "What if???" Thank you, Tom, for opening the conversation. I'm grateful for the patience and encouragement of my husband, Jeff Crosby, who continues to support and is first cheerleader for anything I write, and who upgraded my little pocket camera as a surprise for this book project. I'm also grateful to Dustin and Gillian Crosby; Jennifer and Nino Buono; and my six grandchildren—Ellie, Jack, Tony, Anna, Emily, and Margaret—who continue to help me see new epiphanies in the natural world whenever we hike together. This book is for them, and for the other children of their generation who I hope will grow up to see tallgrass prairie as beautiful, complex, and irreplaceable.